MEDICAL RADIOLOGY

Diagnostic Imaging and Radiation Oncology

Intraoperative Radiotherapy

Clinical Experiences and Results

Contributors

O. Abuchaibe · F. Aguilera · J. Alvarez-Cienfuegos · S. Amillo · J. Aristu · J.L. Arroyo
I. Azinovic · J.L. Beguiristain · J. M. Berián · L.W. Brady · F. A. Calvo · J. Cañadell
F. Carrascosa · F. de la Fuente · L. Escudé · R. García-Tapia · J. L. Hernández
J. Herreros · M. Jurado · R. Llorens · D. Ortiz de Urbina · F. Pardo · M. Santos
J. M. Serra · L. Sierrasesúmaga · E. Tangco · V. Vanaclocha · C.Villas · J. Voltas
G. Zornoza · J. Zudiare

Edited by

Felipe A. Calvo, Manuel Santos, and Luther W. Brady

Foreword by

Luther W. Brady and Hans-Peter Heilmann

Springer-Verlag
Berlin Heidelberg New York
London Paris Tokyo
Hong Kong Barcelona
Budapest

Dr. Felipe Angel Calvo
Director and Consultant

Dr. Manuel Santos
Service of Radiotherapy
Department of Oncology
Clinica Universitaria
E-31080 Pamplona
Spain

Luther W. Brady
Professor and Chairman
Department of Radiation Oncology
Hahnemann University
Broad & Vine, Mail Stop 200
Philadelphia, PA 19102-1192
USA

MEDICAL RADIOLOGY · Diagnostic Imaging and Radiation Oncology
Continuation of
Handbuch der medizinischen Radiologie
Encyclopedia of Medical Radiology

With 60 Figures

ISBN 3-540-52544-0 Springer-Verlag Berlin Heidelberg New York
ISBN 0-387-52544-0 Springer-Verlag New York Berlin Heidelberg

Library of Congress Cataloging-in-Publication Data. Intraoperative radiotherapy : clinical experience and results / contributors, O. Abuchaibe ... [et al.] ; edited by Felipe A. Calvo, Manuel Santos, and Luther W. Brady ; foreword by Luther W. Brady and Hans-Peter Heilmann. p. cm. - (Medical radiology) Includes bibliographical references and index.
ISBN 3-540-52544-0 (alk. paper) ISBN 0-387-52544-0 (alk. paper)
1. Cancer-Intraoperative radiotherapy. I. Abuchaibe, O. II. Calvo, Felipe A. (Felipe Angel). III. Santos, Manuel. IV. Brady, Luther W., 1925- . V. Series.
[DNLM: 1. Intraoperative Care. 2. Neoplasms-radiotherapy. 3. Neoplasms-surgery. QZ 269 I 585] RC 652.I 58 1992
616.99′40642-dc 20 DNLM/DLC

Typesetting: Best-set Typesetter Ltd., Hong Kong
Printing: Appl, Wemding; Bookbinding: J. Schäffer GmbH & Co. K. G., Grünstadt
10/3130-5 4 3 2 1 0 - Printed on acid-free paper

Dedication

to our families

Foreword

The development of the capacity to use electron beams at various energies stimulated the development of the new technology of intraoperative radiation therapy. The visualization of the primary tumor, definition of the site to be irradiated, and knowledge of the size of tumor to be irradiated, including adequate margins for microscopic extent along with debulking of the tumor, have allowed intraoperative radiation therapy to be pursued in a wide variety of disease processes. Not only is it possible to treat tumors that were highly resistant, but it is also possible to specifically localize the tumor with a margin adequate to encompass potential microscopic extensions and to choose the appropriate electron beam energy to treat the potential residual tumor and spare the adjacent normal structures. It is, furthermore, possible to treat patients with unresectable tumors. Central to this entire development is the fact that normal structures can be removed from the field of treatment.

In the beginning, the emphasis was on single fractions of electron beam radiation without subsequent supplementation by external photon beam radiation therapy. However, more recently it has become necessary to use not only a single electron beam fraction during the course of the operation, but to supplement it with external beam treatment.

The encouraging results obtained with intraoperative radiation therapy have led to clinical trials at a large number of institutions throughout the world. To date, more than 4000 patients have been treated using intraoperative radiation therapy with and without supplemental external beam treatment. The increasing enthusiasm for the application of this procedure has resulted in increased expertise in the utilization of the technology.

The present volume represents the experiencc gathered at a single institution in using intraoperative radiation therapy in a wide variety of tumor sites. The various chapters summarize the innovative characteristics of intraoperative radiation therapy in the treatment of patients with malignant disease and describe how this treatment regimen permits improved local/regional control and causes markedly diminished normal tissue toxicities.

LUTHER W. BRADY

HANS-PETER HEILMANN

Preface

Intraoperative radiotherapy (IORT) is an experimental cancer treatment modality that permits the delivery of a high single dose of radiation (ideally using electron beams) in a surgically defined area, while normal uninvolved tissues surrounding the target area are mobilized or protected from radiation. IORT is, then, a modality to intensify locoregional treatment and promote high local tumor control rates, and/or to decrease the normal tissue toxicity from conventional treatment. IORT is in this context an attractive treatment modality because it brings together two classic forms of cancer therapy with well-established results: surgery and radiotherapy. Improved cooperation between surgeons and radiation oncologists will always produce positive results in cancer treatment, and IORT is the type of program that requires serious consideration by groups active in clinical research. The development of an IORT program in any institution is a small revolution.

The complexity of personnel coordination and technical requirements might discourage physicians and their associates at the early stages of the program. IORT needs a peculiar sense of discipline among the physicians responsible for the different protocols. The technique itself has to be as simple and as fast as possible. The professional involved in IORT has to realize that it represents simultaneously an extra effort to improve prognosis in cancer patients with an unfavorable outlook and a means of answering important scientific questions in developmental therapeutic research.

This monograph is a review of the clinical experiences and results obtained with IORT in a single European institution over a period of 5 years. The data are presented in a synthetic way to emphasize the fact that cooperation among specialists can produce a significant amount of information. At the present time the treatment programs tested might serve as baseline phase I–II clinical trials in tumors of multiple sites. The development of more sophisticated and scientifically meaningful programs, such as phase II–III or phase III trials, will depend upon cooperation among expert institutions and groups. As more centers gain the appropriate skills in IORT, and as more refined criteria and techniques are developed, it is reasonable to hope that IORT will come to render anecdotal the term "local recurrence." Local and regional control are the ultimate aim of surgery and radiotherapy in clinical oncology.

FELIPE A. CALVO
MANUEL SANTOS
LUTHER W. BRADY

Acknowledgments

Upon completion of a book it is natural for authors to feel a need to express gratitude to the persons who made their work possible, and in the field of multidisciplinary oncology the omission of such an acknowledgment would be particularly unjust. The results that are available for analysis have been acquired through the effort and professional excellence of many physicians, nurses, and health personnel. Furthermore the treatment modality that is the subject of this monograph, namely intraoperative radiotherapy (IORT), demands of those involved unusually high levels of enthusiasm, imagination, and intellectual interest, as well as the best loving patient care. During the period over which the clinical experiences referred to in this book were gained, more than 100 people were involved directly in patient care. Their names will not appear in the text, but they are written in some silent page of the book of Medicine. Here, it must suffice to make general mention of the Departments closely involved in IORT: Anesthesia, Surgery, Neurosurgery, Otorhinolaryngology, Plastic and Reconstructive Surgery, Cardiovascular and Thoracic Surgery, Urology, Gynecology and Obstetrics, Orthopedic Surgery and Traumatology, and the Pediatric Oncology Unit. To all of them our deep gratitude.

Separatc mention has to be made of the operating room and radiotherapy nurses, who in the period 1984–1989 were Milagros Arrieta (supervisor), María Angeles Aznarez, Ana Elzaburu, María José Gil, Pilar Imizcoz, Blanca E. Leache, Rosario Moreno, Concha Soriano, and Manuela Villena. Their dedication to this particular treatment modality has been reflected in a creativity which has improved many aspects of the procedure and also the quality of patients' safety, comfort, and ultimately medical care.

In addition, thanks should be expressed to our colleagues in the Division of Medical Oncology for their open attitude towards the integration of a novel treatment modality in the management of cancer patients.

The principal editor (F. A. C.) wishes to thank the secretaries of the Department of Oncology, María Carmen Lacosta, Begoña Lezano, and Rosario Pacheco, for their quiet and constant support in the preparation of the manuscript, and Dr. Enrico Tangco for his generous and meticulous work in assisting the editor.

Contents

1 Intraoperative Radiotherapy: Rationale and Program Development
FELIPE A. CALVO, MANUEL SANTOS, and LUTHER W. BRADY 1

2 Physics
LLUIS ESCUDÉ, DAVID ORTIZ DE URBINA, and ENRICO TANGCO 11

3 Anesthesia and Hospital Coordination
DAVID ORTIZ DE URBINA, ENRICO TANGCO, JOSÉ LUIS ARROYO, and FRANCISCO CARRASCOSA 25

4 Intracranial Tumors
FELIPE A. CALVO, OSCAR ABUCHAIBE, VICENTE VANACLOCHA, and FRANCISCO AGUILERA 31

5 Head and Neck Cancer
FELIPE A. CALVO, OSCAR ABUCHAIBE, JOSÉ MARÍA SERRA, and RAFAEL GARCÍA-TAPIA 37

6 Lung Cancer
FELIPE A. CALVO, DAVID ORTIZ DE URBINA, JESÚS HERREROS, and RAFAEL LLORENS 43

7 Gastric Cancer
FELIPE A. CALVO, MANUEL SANTOS, FERNANDO PARDO, JOSÉ L. HERNÁNDEZ, JAVIER ALVAREZ-CIENFUEGOS, and JUAN VOLTAS 51

8 Pancreatic Cancer
FELIPE A. CALVO, IGNACIO AZINOVIC, GERARDO ZORNOZA, JUAN VOLTAS, FERNANDO PARDO, and JAVIER ALVAREZ-CIENFUEGOS 57

9 Colorectal Cancer
FELIPE A. CALVO, IGNACIO AZINOVIC, FERNANDO PARDO, JOSÉ L. HERNÁNDEZ, and JAVIER ALVAREZ-CIENFUEGOS 65

10 Bladder Cancer
FELIPE A. CALVO, OSCAR ABUCHAIBE, JAVIER ARISTU, JAVIER ZUDIARE, and JOSÉ MARÍA BERIÁN 73

11 Gynecologic Cancer
FELIPE A. CALVO, DAVID ORTIZ DE URBINA, FERNANDO DE LA FUENTE, MATIAS JURADO, and JOSÉ MARÍA BERIÁN 79

12 Retroperitoneal and Other Central Soft Tissue Sarcomas
Felipe A. Calvo, Oscar Abuchaibe, José María Serra, José María Berián, and José Cañadell 85

13 Soft Tissue Sarcomas of the Extremities
Felipe A. Calvo, David Ortiz de Urbina, José L. Beguiristain, Santiago Amillo, and José Cañadell 91

14 Ewing's Sarcoma
Felipe A. Calvo, Oscar Abuchaibe, Carlos Villas, José Cañadell, and Luis Sierrasesúmaga 99

15 Osteosarcoma
Felipe A. Calvo, Ignacio Azinovic, Santiago Amillo, José Cañadell, and Luis Sierrasesúmaga 103

16 Summary and Future Prospects
Felipe A. Calvo, Manuel Santos, and Luther W. Brady 109

Subject Index 115

List of Contributors 117

1 Intraoperative Radiotherapy: Rationale and Program Development

FELIPE A. CALVO, MANUEL SANTOS, and LUTHER W. BRADY

CONTENTS

1.1 Definition . . . 1
1.2 Rationale: Improving the Therapeutic Index . . 1
1.2.1 Geographic Miss Rate . . . 1
1.2.2 Normal Tissue Toxicity . . . 2
1.2.3 Biologic Efficacy of Radiation Therapy . . . 2
1.3 Integration in Multidisciplinary Oncology . . . 2
1.3.1 IORT and Surgery . . . 2
1.3.2 IORT and External Beam Radiotherapy . . . 3
1.3.3 IORT and Radiation Modifiers . . . 3
1.4 Clinical Trials . . . 3
1.4.1 Protocol Design . . . 3
1.4.2 Quality Control Parameters . . . 4
1.4.3 Assessment of Tumor Response . . . 5
1.4.4 Local Tumor Control Analysis . . . 6
1.5 General Considerations Regarding the Clinical Experience at the Clinica Universitaria de Navarra . . . 7
1.5.1 Study Design . . . 8
1.5.2 Tumor Sites . . . 8
1.5.3 Histologic Types . . . 9
References . . . 9

1.1 Definition

Since ionizing radiation is used for the treatment of malignant disease, several methods have been developed to deliver radiation treatment during a surgical intervention. Interstitial implantation of different radio isotopes is a valuable technique used for selected indications in modern radiation oncology (PEREZ and GLASGOW 1987). The increasing interest in intraoperative electron beam irradiation in recent decades requires a restatement of its rationale. There is a consensus among oncologists that intraoperative radiation therapy (IORT) is a treatment technique in which a high single dose of fast electrons is delivered in a surgically defined area, while trying to protect normal tissues from the radiation beam (either by retracting the mobile structures or by shielding the fixed ones).

Historically IORT was first performed using primitive low energy x-rays (BECK 1907). The development of new technology for radiation therapy made available beams of fast electrons for clinical practice. The pioneers of modern IORT immediately adopted this form of radiation due to its physical properties and the dosimetric advantages (ABE 1989).

1.2 Rationale: Improving the Therapeutic Index

Intraoperative radiation therapy is a technique developed to improve the therapeutic index by the combination of surgery and radiation therapy in the treatment of cancer patients. The therapeutic index in clinical oncology, and particularly in radiation oncology, is related to the antitumor activity of the particular treatment approach, together with the tolerance of normal tissues. Conventional cancer surgery and radiotherapy, and the combination of both modalities, appear to have reached a plateau in achieving local tumor control. IORT might improve the therapeutic index by reducing the geographic miss rate and the normal tissue toxicity of external beam radiotherapy, or by increasing the biologic efficacy of radiation therapy.

1.2.1 Geographic Miss Rate

During cancer surgery the tumor, areas of residual disease, and high risk zones for recurrence can be accurately delineated for IORT. This has a

FELIPE A. CALVO, Dr., Director and Consultant, MANUEL SANTOS, Dr., Radiotherapy Division, Department of Oncology, Clinica Universitaria de Navarra, 31080 Pamplona, Spain

LUTHER W. BRADY, MD, Professor and Chairman, Hahnemann University, Department of Radiation Oncology and Nuclear Medicine, Broad & Vine, Mail Stop 200, Philadelphia, PA 19102-1192, USA positive effect on the therapeutic index of the combined treatment approach by decreasing the geographic miss rate of conventional external beam radiotherapy. Even with the vast improvements made in diagnostic imaging and their incorporation in expert systems for radiation therapy planning, visualization of the treatment area at the time of surgery remains the most reliable means of tumor definition.

1.2.2 Normal Tissue Toxicity

As already mentioned, mobile structures and organs can be displaced from the radiation beam in most anatomic zones, while fixed structures can occasionally be protected by shielding if necessary. These techniques can be applied to many structures and organs, e.g., small bowel, lung, and ureters. However, while it is in general true that both techniques will decrease the normal tissue toxicity in IORT programs, in recent years it has emerged that certain tissues which are either immobile or unsuitable for shielding, e.g., peripheral nerves and major blood vessels, limit the size of the single fractions of electrons that can be employed (Kinsella et al. 1984). As a consequence a compromise must be reached in selecting the IORT dose.

1.2.3 Biologic Efficacy of Radiation Therapy

There is controversy in basic radiobiology regarding the biologic effect of high single fractions of radiation delivered to tumor tissue (Dobelbower 1989). Nevertheless, the current tendency is to use IORT as a boosting technique in combination with conventional fractionated external beam irradiation. This approach maintains the advantages of fractionation in radiotherapy, and the total dose delivered to the target volume is in many instances far superior to that which can be achieved with sophisticated external beam radiotherapy techniques alone.

One factor that can improve the therapeutic index in IORT trials is tumor resection. Thus it has been reported that tumor control increases in correlation with the excellence of the tumor resection in IORT trials (Tepper et al. 1984; Sindelar and Kinsella 1986). When resection is possible, most hypoxic cells will be removed and IORT will treat a small amount of residual disease or an area at high risk for recurrence. These peripheral tumor cells are thought to be well oxygenated, proliferating, and in cell cycle phases sensitive to radiation effects.

1.3 Integration in Multidisciplinary Oncology

1.3.1 IORT and Surgery

Intraoperative radiation therapy is a modality that cannot be developed without strong support from surgical oncology (Sindelar et al. 1988). The program is based on an understanding among radiotherapists and surgeons of the possibilities and limitations of cancer surgery, IORT, conventional external beam radiotherapy, and tumor behavior. Initially, IORT was used for intra-abdominal tumors due to the evident improvement in the delineation of areas involved by tumor and the protection of dose-limiting organs and structures. Most IORT protocols have explored this combined approach in locally advanced neoplasms in spite of the inconveniences, difficulties, and complications related to extensive surgical procedures in patients with advanced cancer. Special care should be offered to these patients during the surgical–IORT procedure and in the postoperative period. This is mandatory to obtain meaningful long-term therapeutic information. In the design of surgical–IORT studies in patients with advanced and/or recurrent disease, tumor resection should be stressed. Surgical incisions can be modified in such a way as to ensure that the exposure of the involved area, the positioning of the IORT cone, and the mobilization of normal organs and structures are achieved in a simple, safe, fast, and uncomplicated manner. Before the patient is moved to the treatment room, adequate hemostasis should be achieved, and it is useful to simulate the mobilization of normal structures in the operating room. The surgeon should define those organs and structures involved by or adjacent to the tumor or tumor bed that cannot be protected from the radiation beam (duodenum, peripheral nerves, large vessels, ureters, etc.). It is important to discuss with the anesthesiologist the status of the patient in order to avoid exposing the patient to any increased risk following hypotensive or arrhythmic episodes during the surgical procedure. Extensive pelvic surgery, in particular, requires close cooperation between radiotherapists and surgeons owing to the technical difficulties in tumor resection, hemostasis, IORT cone positioning, sparing of normal tissues, and postoperative patient care.

1.3.2 IORT and External Beam Radiotherapy

Recent data in IORT have been generated using IORT as a boosting modality combined with conventional programs of fractionated external beam radiotherapy (Gunderson et al. 1983, 1984). This approach permits the exploitation of the biologic advantages of fractionation in radiotherapy, together with the use of large treatment volumes that include the primary tumor site and nodal draining zones, while the surgical area is boosted with a single large fraction of electrons (10–20 Gy). Preoperative external beam radiotherapy seems interesting for those tumors or tumor sites for which advantages in tumor resectability have been reported (e.g., rectosigmoid carcinoma). Nevertheless, if the patient is referred first to a surgical team it will be uncommon to have the opportunity to offer preoperative radiotherapy.

Those patients with recurrence in a previously irradiated zone pose an interesting and difficult problem. In many instances these patients have had pelvic primaries and are being considered for rescue surgery. In these cases IORT can be used to treat tumor bed areas. High single doses of radiation are selected (20–25 Gy), and large treatment cones recommended. Obviously, generally such patients have a poor prognosis and are exposed to major complications from the surgical procedure and IORT. It should be mentioned that a small and selected group of patients with head and neck and soft tissue sarcomas have been treated using myocutaneous flaps to cover the postsurgical skin defect. With this new tissue in the area of treatment some additional external beam radiotherapy can be delivered to the zone.

1.3.3 IORT and Radiation Modifiers

Intraoperative radiation therapy can be explored in conjunction with different radiation modifiers such as chemotherapeutic agents, radiation sensitizers, and hyperthermia. The fact that IORT is given in a short period of time and to a confined anatomic area offers an attractive biologic human model in the search for modifiers of radiation damage in human tumor tissue. Initial reports have shown the feasibility of developing this investigational approach (Tepper et al. 1987; Merrick et al. 1987).

In general, systemic chemotherapy should be maintained in those cases in which it is considered an important part of the disease management. A special effort has to be made to develop effective chemotherapy regimes in diseases with a high risk of distant metastasis when treating locally advanced tumor stages and/or local recurrences. IORT will only improve local tumor control rates, and its value might not be appreciated if systemic failures are common.

1.4 Clinical Trials

1.4.1 Protocol Design

Developmental therapeutics in clinical oncology involve a continual search for ways of improving the quality of therapy in cancer patients. Research regarding conventional treatment modalities for cancer – surgery, radiotherapy, and chemotherapy – is directed towards the development of new approaches to increase antitumor efficacy. In recent decades a major effort has been made to design combined treatment protocols that will optimize technique and improve results in the multidisciplinary management of cancer patients.

In recent years IORT has been receiving increasing attention in clinical oncology (Dobelbower and Abe 1989). Although IORT is considered an investigational treatment procedure, most experts in the field would probably agree that IORT is feasible in multiple anatomic areas. Acute and long-term complications are being assessed in carefully designed experimental and clinical studies. Physics and quality control parameters are being established in the different programs. Prospective multi-institutional trials have been activated, accomplishing a final important step in clinical trial design. Figure 1.1 depicts coordination requirements for the development of IORT trials (Calvo and Hanks 1988).

Initially, IORT has to be tested as a developmental therapeutic modality in phase I–II oriented trials. Although a large amount of information is available on the feasibility of IORT and its most common toxicities and complications,

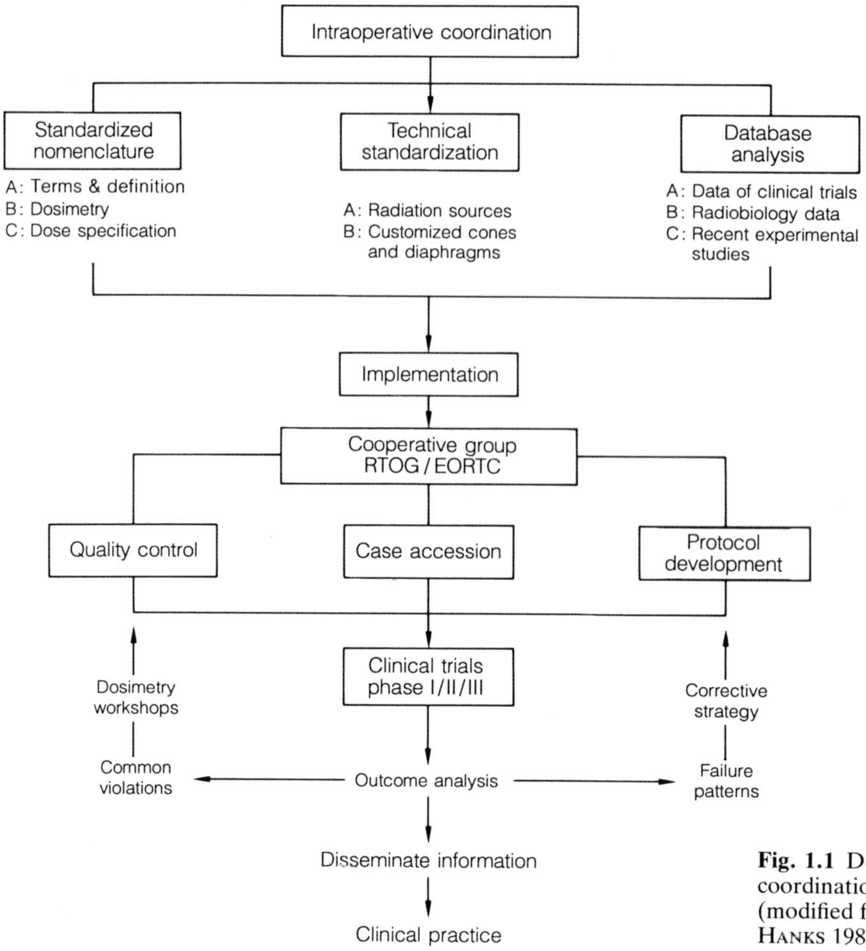

Fig. 1.1 Development and coordination of IORT trials (modified from CALVO and HANKS 1988)

each institutional program has to reproduce comparable data before prospective phase III comparative studies can be activated. The objectives and specific aims of IORT trials are summarized below:

Objectives:
- Demonstrate efficacy
- Identify normal tissue toxicity
- Demonstrate the advantage over the best current management in selected diseases
- Identify adjuvants (hypoxic cell sensitizers, chemotherapy) that may improve effectiveness
- Determine the optimal sequencing of surgical resection, IORT, sensitizers or chemotherapy, and external beam treatment

Specific Aims:
- Conduct phase II clinical trials in a spectrum of disease sites where the use of IORT is logically justified
- Conduct prospective randomized trials in sites selected from those tested, comparing IORT with the best current management
- Conduct phase I–II trials testing toxicity and efficacy of hypoxic cell sensitizers and selected chemotherapeutic agents in combination with IORT
- Introduce chemotherapy sensitizers in prospective random trials as indicated by the above phase I–II trials

1.4.2 Quality Control Parameters

Quality assurance in IORT is based on comparative analysis of the data available on physical and dosimetric aspects, animal studies on normal tissue tolerance with or without surgical manipulation, and observations regarding toxicity and complications in ongoing clinical trials. A report published by US investigators from various institutions has tabulated clinical observations of interest for the analysis of quality control parameters in IORT trials (Tepper et al. 1986).

In our own institution a written protocol has to be signed by the principal surgeon and radiotherapist involved in each procedure, recording the major facts pertaining to that particular case. The data are collected on the same day as the IORT procedure and contain the following information:

Disease Status:
- Tumor site
- Tumor histology
- Tumor stage
- Previous treatment(s)

Surgery:
- Type of operation
- Definition of the anatomic zone involved in treatment
- Residual disease (macroscopic or microscopic) after surgery
- Name of the principal surgeon

Radiotherapy:
- Cone size (diameter in cm)
- Beveled angle (0°, 15°, 30°, 45°)
- Source–tumor distance (cm)
- Electron energy selected (MeV)
- Total single dose (Gy)
- Single/multiple field (overlaps)
- Structures included in the field (sutures)
- Structures mobilized out of the field
- Structures shielded in the field
- Gantry angulation
- Polaroid photograph or video taping of the procedure
- Special features during IORT: hemorrhage, etc.
- Physics calculations of monitor units
- Name of the principal radiotherapist

Anesthesia:
- Transportation time
- Treatment time
- Duration of the surgical procedure (including the IORT component)
- Drugs administered
- Blood transfusion
- Major ECG and blood pressure abnormalities (arrhythmias, hypotensive episodes)
- Name of the principal anesthesiologist

It has proven convenient to have notes regarding the postoperative period as a special part of the clinical records of patients treated with IORT. Patients who have entered the IORT program should also be entered in a database system including patient, tumor, and treatment characteristics. In the follow-up period, toxicities and complications, patterns of tumor recurrence, and patient status should be noted and updated.

1.4.3 Assessment of Tumor Response

Unresected or partially resected tumors are candidates for tumor response evaluation if there is pre- and postoperative documentation of tumor location, size, and extension. Computed tomography (CT) and magnetic resonance imaging (MRI) are most useful means of assessing tumor response following IORT. Pancreatic cancer is a good example for the evaluation of tumor response. In general the primary lesion does not change in size, or only minor changes are noticeable. In patients who have achieved long-term survival (more than 10–12 months), no increase in tumor size can be noted even when distant metastases have developed. In a proportion of patients the follow-up period will be short to establish tumor response. Advanced or recurrent rectosigmoid cancer also serves to highlight some of the difficulties inherent in assessing tumor response in IORT patients. In the pelvic area, postsurgical changes are the rule following extensive procedures, and postoperative CT can be used to show a presacral mass compatible with hematoma, fibrosis, or persistent and/or recurrent tumor. The initial postoperative CT scan might serve as a baseline image in the follow-up of such patients. Some of them will eventually develop pelvic pain, and differential diagnosis between tumor progression and neuropathy may be difficult. In unresectable lung cancer, tumor response can be well documented (Figs. 1.2, 1.3), but late lung parenchymal changes will again cause diagnostic problems as to whether tumor progression or fibrosis is developing (Fig. 1.4).

Protocols in which organ or tumor removal is performed following IORT and external beam radiotherapy (in our institution this is done in the case of deep invasive bladder cancer) represent exceptions to the norm. In such protocols tumor response is documented by the study of the tissues removed.

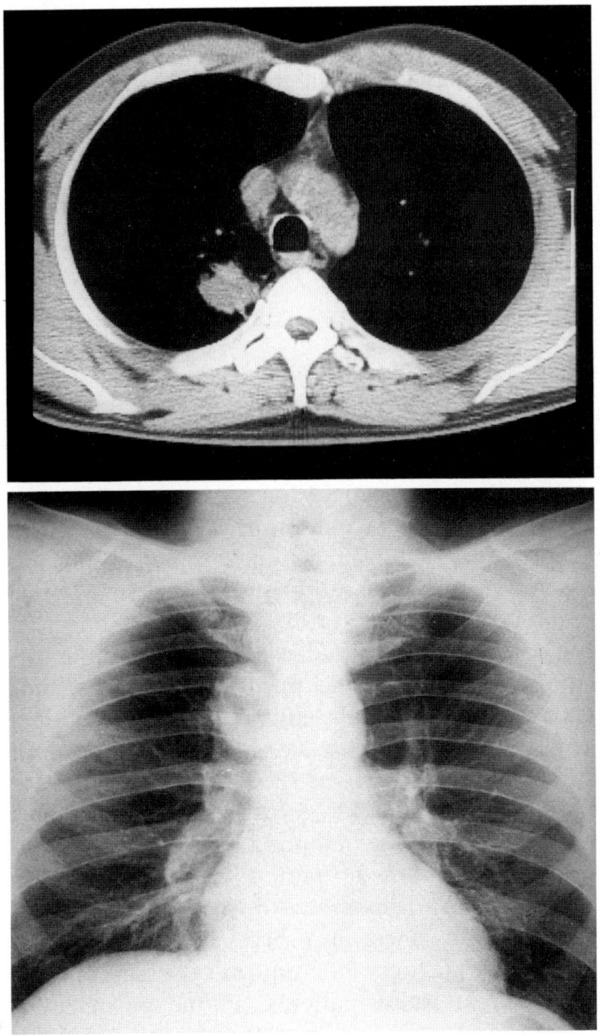

a

b

Fig. 1.2a,b. Unresectable adenocarcinoma of the right upper lobe. The patient was treated with 10 Gy IORT (20 MeV electrons) and 46 Gy external beam irradiation. **a** CT scan; **b** chest x-ray. Images before treatment

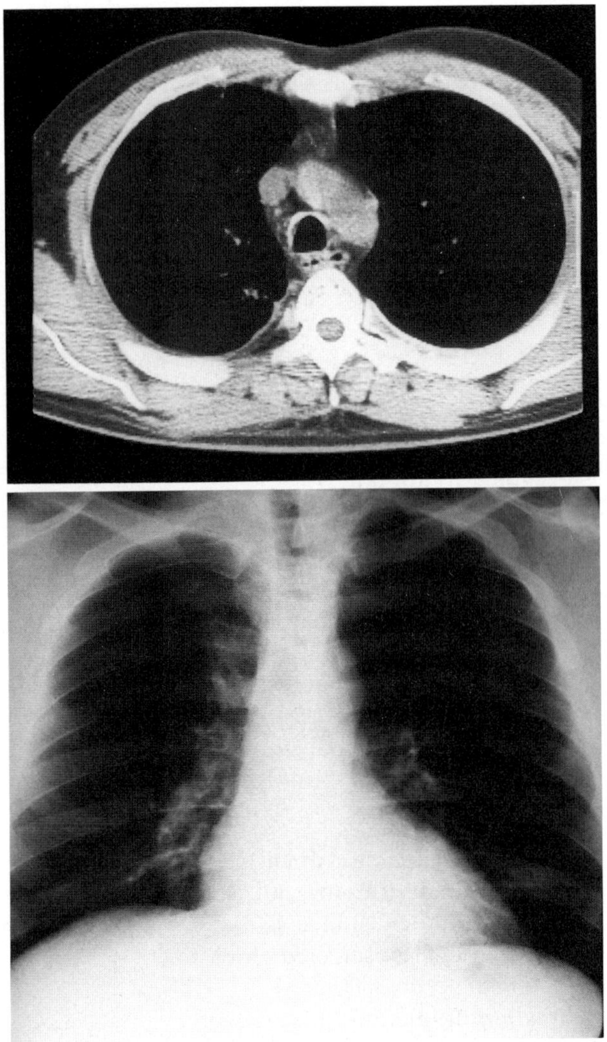

a

b

Fig. 1.3a,b. Case illustrated in Fig. 1.2, a few months after the completion of radiotherapy. Tumor remission is documented by **a** CT and **b** chest x-ray

1.4.4 Local Tumor Control Analysis

Patterns of tumor relapse should be carefully monitored in IORT protocols. It is important to obtain this information in IORT studies because of the high local tumor control rates expected from this modality in selected tumor sites. The patterns of relapse will aid the development of new treatment strategies as well as providing insight into how to modify surgery, IORT, and external beam radiotherapy so as to intensify locoregional treatment programs.

1.4.4.1 Importance and Contribution of IORT Programs in Locoregional Tumor Control

Within the contemporary context of multidisciplinary oncology, the potential contribution of IORT is to increase local tumor control rates in multiple tumor sites. Surgery and radiotherapy have been employed together for a long time, and a plateau in local control rates has consequently been reached. Furthermore, locally advanced tumors impose limitations on both surgical resection and external beam irradiation. A relevant concern in this type of disease presentation is systemic dissemination at the time of diagnosis,

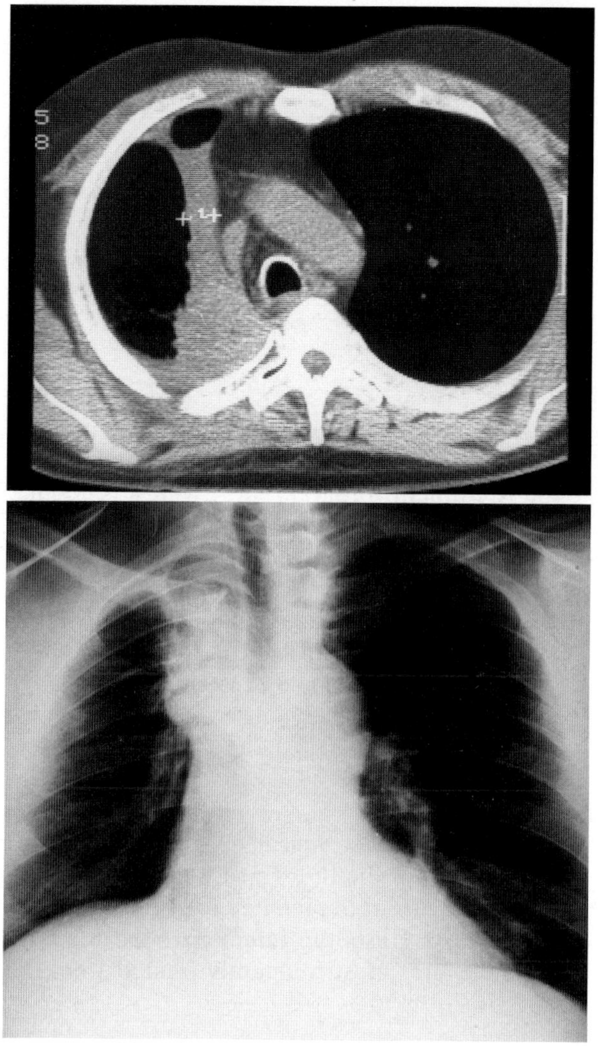

a

b

Fig. 1.4a,b. Long-term changes in the area of the initial primary lesion. Images (**a** CT scan; **b** chest x-ray) obtained 35 months after IORT

and even if we are able to increase local control rates with IORT, patients will be lost due to the development of distant metastases. Therefore adjuvant chemotherapy should be incorporated in IORT programs in accordance with the tumor site, histology, efficacy, and availability.

Cooperation among investigators involved in IORT should be stressed. Rapid accrual of clinical information pertaining to recurrent and/or advanced malignant disease may permit the use of this modality in early tumor stages, in which various benefits in the management of cancer patients, such as decreased toxicity and improvement of local tumor control and/or survival rates, may be possible. Tumor types never previously tested might also be considered for IORT protocols.

Therapeutic programs that increase local control rates in human cancer represent an improvement in the quality of therapy and the quality of life. Such improvement is one of the objectives of IORT. Increases in survival will only be detected in early disease stages or in patients with tumors that have a low tendency for systemic dissemination.

1.5 General Considerations Regarding the Clinical Experience at the Clinica Universitaria de Navarra

The activation of the IORT program in the Department of Oncology was initially presented to our surgical colleagues as the clinical research priority of the Radiotherapy Division. The modality was introduced as a treatment intensification technique in which a high single fraction boost of radiotherapy was delivered to unresectable or partially resected tumors. The advantage of protecting normal tissues was particularly attractive. Information regarding technical aspects, literature on normal tissue tolerance, and clinical data were disseminated among the different surgical departments involved in cancer surgery. As soon as the IORT procedure was proved to be fast, safe, and easy to perform, an increased number of patients were considered candidates for IORT. The constant support given by our surgical colleagues, and particularly the anesthesiologist, made possible the investigation of IORT in multiple tumor sites and different histologic types. The treatment protocols were phase I–II oriented studies. There was a consensus among both surgeons and radiotherapists on the major aspects of the combined treatment program: type of surgery, IORT volume definition and dose delivered, and the external beam component of the treatment. Positive clinical signs were soon noticed in patients treated with IORT, such as relief of abdominal pain in pancreatic cancer and tumor remission in lung cancer. The tolerance of normal tissues was acceptable, with no increase in postoperative complications. These facts, plus the observation of high local control rates within the treated area, led to the adoption of a rather systematic approach in patients undergoing cancer surgery.

Enough data are now available to support new strategies or the development of phase III trials. These efforts should be made in collaboration with other institutions owing to the limited number of patients that each protocol can reach in any particular institution in a reasonable period of time.

1.5.1 Study Design

The following factors influenced the selection of tumor sites for investigation in our institution:

- The available information of possible relevance to the use of IORT in the management of tumors of various sites
- The willingness of the surgical departments to collaborate in the use of IORT
- Miscellaneous considerations pertaining to the use of IORT in patients with locally advanced disease or tumor recurrences

In those tumor sites where close cooperation from the surgeons assured good accrual of patients, the study was defined as a phase I–II trial in which the final end points were technical feasibility, prospective evaluation of toxicity and complications, and local tumor control analysis. Survival data were always available to any investigator involved in the program.

The general features of the treatment protocols were:

- Maximal surgical tumor resection.
- IORT with moderate doses (20 Gy for unresected tumors, 15 Gy for gross residual disease, 10 Gy for microscopic or high risk areas). The treatment cone had to include the lesion plus at least a 1-cm margin of normal tissue. The electron energy selected had to include the area of disease with a margin (at least 0.5–1 cm) in the 90% isodose curve.
- External beam radiotherapy with conventional fields including the primary lesion and nodal drainage areas, and conventional fractionation (1.8–2 Gy daily, five times per week), reaching doses of 46–50 Gy. This modality was omitted in osteosarcomas, most pediatric cases, and in patients with recurrences in a previously irradiated zone. In Ewing's sarcoma and some bronchogenic and colorectal carcinoma patients external beam radiotherapy was given preoperatively.

Table 1.1. Tumor sites treated with IORT (1984–1989)

Tumor site	No. of procedures	%
Intracranial	12	2
Head and neck	24	4
Intrathoracic	75	15
Intra-abdominal		
Upper abdomen	131	26
Pelvis	114	22
Extremities	121	24
Miscellaneous	21	4
Total	498	100

- Systemic adjuvant or neoadjuvant treatment. Chemotherapy is an important component of the treatment program in Ewing's sarcoma, osteosarcoma, high grade soft tissue sarcomas, and some other miscellaneous tumors (lymphomas, Wilms' tumor, etc.). More recently, chemotherapy has been included in a neoadjuvant investigational fashion in the management of lung, bladder, and colorectal carcinoma.

1.5.2 Tumor Sites

The analysis of the clinical experience obtained includes many of the IORT procedures performed in the period from September 1984 to December 1989. Table 1.1 lists the tumor sites treated with IORT; the sites most frequently treated were the

Table 1.2. Histologic distribution of tumor types treated with IORT (1984–1989)

Histology/site	No. of patients	%
Lung cancer	72	15
Bone sarcomas	62	12
Soft tissue sarcomas	59	11
Colorectal cancer	54	10
Gastric cancer	45	8
Pancreatic cancer	49	9
Gynecologic cancer	26	5
Bladder cancer	30	5
Renal carcinoma	23	4
Head and neck cancer	15	3
Miscellaneous	15	3
Melanoma	7	2
Retroperitoneal sarcoma	6	1
Wilms' tumor	4	1
Lymphoma	4	1
Prostatic cancer	4	1
Cholangiocarcinoma	2	1
Neuroblastoma	2	1
Total	491	100

extremities and intra-abdominal and intrathoracic sites.

1.5.3 Histologic Types

The distribution of histologic types is listed in Table 1.2. It seems evident that the tumors treated do not follow epidemiologic data, with the possible exception of lung cancer: the number of patients with a particular histology treated by IORT has more to do with the requirements stated in the initial IORT protocols. On the other hand, previously established programs, such as preservation of extremities in cases of bone and soft tissue sarcoma, attracted a significant number of patients to our institution, which made it possible to explore IORT in these tumor subtypes.

References

Abe M (1989) History of intraoperative radiation therapy. In: Dobelbower RR, Abe M (eds) Intraoperative radiation therapy. CRC, Boca Raton, Fl, pp 1–10

Beck C (1907) Über Kombinationsbehandlung bei bösartigen Neubildunqen. Berl Klin Wochenschr 44: 1335

Calvo FA, Hanks GE (1988) Intraoperative trials. Int J Radiat Oncol Biol Phys 14: S111–S117

Dobelbower RR (1989) The rationale for intraoperative radiotherapy. In: Dobelbower RR, Abe M (eds) Intraoperative radiation therapy. CRC, Boca Raton, Fl, pp 11–16

Dobelbower RR, Abe M (1989) Intraoperative radiation therapy. CRC, Boca Raton, Fl

Gunderson LL, Cohen AC, Dosoretz DD et al. (1983) Residual, unresectable, or recurrent colorectal cancer: external beam irradiation and intraoperative electron boost + resection. Int J Radiat Oncol Biol Phys 9: 1597–1606

Gunderson LL, Martin NK, Earle JD et al. (1984) Intraoperative and external beam irradiation with or without resection: Mayo pilot experience. Mayo Clin Proc 59: 691–699

Kinsella TJ, Sindelar WF, de Luca AM, Terrill R (1984) Tolerance of peripheral nerve to intraoperative radiotherapy (IORT): clinical and experimental studies. Int J Radiat Oncol Biol Phys 10: 80–84

Merrick HW, Milligan AJ, Woldenberg LS et al. (1987) Intraoperative interstitial hyperthermia in conjunction with intraoperative radiation therapy in a radiation-resistant carcinoma of the abdomen: report on the feasibility of a new technique. J Surg Oncol 36: 48–51

Perez CA, Glasgow CP (1987) Clinical applications of brachytherapy. In: Perez CA, Brady LW (eds) Principles and practice of radiation oncology. JB Lippincott, Philadelphia, pp 252–290

Sindelar WF, Kinsella TJ (1986) Randomized trial of intraoperative radiotherapy in resected carcinoma of the pancreas. Int J Radiat Oncol Biol Phys 12 [Suppl 1]: 148

Sindelar WF, Hoekstra HJ, Kinsella TJ (1988) Surgical approaches and techniques in intraoperative radiotherapy for intra-abdominal retroperitoneal and pelvic neoplasms. Surgery 103: 247–256

Tepper JE, Wood WC, Cohen AM et al. (1984) Intraoperative radiation therapy. In: De Vita VT, Hellman S, Rosenberg SA (eds) Important advances in oncology. JB Lippincott, Philadelphia, pp 226–242

Tepper JE, Gunderson LL, Goldson AL et al. (1986) Quality control parameters of intraoperative radiation therapy. Int J Radiat Oncol Biol Phys 12: 1687–1695

Tepper JE, Shipley WU, Warshaw AL et al. (1987) The role of misonidazole combined with intraoperative radiation therapy in the treatment of pancreatic carcinoma. J Clin Oncol 5: 579–584

2 Physics

LLUIS ESCUDÉ, DAVID ORTIZ DE URBINA, and ENRICO TANGCO

CONTENTS

2.1	Introduction	11
2.2	Characteristics of Electron Beams	11
2.2.1	Depth-Dose Curves	11
2.2.2	Interaction of Radiation with Matter	13
2.2.3	Beam Profiles	14
2.2.4	Isodose Curves	16
2.3	Description of Applicators for External Beam Radiotherapy	17
2.4	Applicators for IORT as Designed at the Clinica Universitaria de Navarra	18
2.5	Dosimetry of IORT Applicators	19
2.5.1	Introduction	19
2.5.2	Output Factors	19
2.5.3	Distance Correction Factors	20
2.5.4	Depth–Dose Data	21
2.5.5	Beam Profiles	21
2.6	Results	22
	References	23

2.1 Introduction

Intraoperative radiotherapy has been made possible by the increasing availability of high energy electron beams to radiation therapy departments. It is true that orthovoltage x-rays were used for this purpose as early as 1905 (BECK 1907, 1909), but only with the ability to generate and handle electron beams with variable energies has IORT begun to be employed as an alternative treatment or as a boosting technique together with external beam radiotherapy.

Electron beams have some physical characteristics that render them different from x-ray and other radiation beams. Special collimating devices, known as applicators, are needed to shape the beam for optimal performance, and these devices are of particular importance for the medical physicist in an IORT program.

LLUIS ESCUDÉ, PhD, Medical Physics Section, DAVID ORTIZ DE URBINA, Dr., ENRICO TANGCO, Dr., Radiotherapy Division, Department of Oncology, Clinica Universitaria de Navarra, 31080 Pamplona, Spain

The design of new applicators especially suited to IORT results in electron beams somewhat different from the regular pattern. This requires from the physics team a whole series of new measurements both to check whether the design yields correct results and to collect data for the records, to be used in treatment planning at later stages.

This chapter first reviews the features of electron beams, comparing them with x-rays; the origin of these features is sought in the behavior of radiation at the atomic level when it interacts with matter. The electron beam collimating devices are then discussed, along with the modifications required for IORT. After comparing the results of calibration with conventional and IORT electron beams, several methods for overcoming some inconveniences are pointed out which result in the design of sophisticated applicators especially suited to IORT.

2.2 Characteristics of Electron Beams

2.2.1 Depth-Dose Curves

The feature that makes electron beams especially suitable for IORT is their typical spatial distribution in human body tissues that results mostly from the way they are attenuated as they travel deeper into these tissues.

The behavior of a radiation beam as it passes through tissue is reflected in the so-called depth-dose curves in which the fractional or percentage (normalized) dose is plotted versus depth, i.e., distance from the beam entrance point at the skin to points inside the patient's body along the central ray of the beam.

Comparison of the typical shapes of the depth-dose curves for the two most common types of radiation available in radiation therapy departments worldwide, photons (x-rays) and electrons, shows at first glance in a qualitative form how the

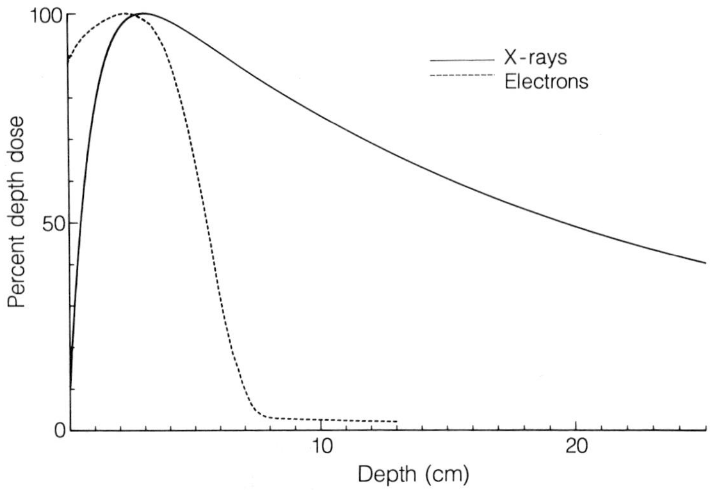

Fig. 2.1. Typical depth–dose curves for a photon beam (*solid line*) and an electron beam (*dashed line*)

energy is deposited at different points. In Fig. 2.1, the absorbed dose, energy absorbed per unit mass, is plotted against depth, for typical electron and photon beams. It can be seen that photons are attenuated at a lower rate than electrons; thus whereas photons deliver a considerable amount of dose deep inside the body, electrons deliver all of their energy in a shallow layer of tissue at a few centimeters beneath the skin, consequently sparing tissues beyond the fall-off zone.

Furthermore, the dose to the entrance surface, normally the skin, is kept low with photon beams but is very high in the case of electron beams. This is one of the latter's few disadvantages in external beam radiotherapy because of possible side-effects on the skin. However, it is rather a desirable effect in IORT since radiation strikes the exposed tumor directly.

Another important feature of high energy photon and electron beams is the fact that the depth at which the maximum absorbed dose occurs is not the entrance point but slightly deeper within the tissue; the higher the beam energy is, the deeper it penetrates. The reason has to do with the fact that absorbed dose in a point in tissue is defined in terms of energy per unit mass imparted at a small volume surrounding that point, which is totally absorbed there. When a radiation beam interacts with matter, whether it consists of photons or electrons, other electrons which are bound to the atoms of the elements constituting the body tissues may receive enough energy from the beam to overcome those energy bonds. When these secondary electrons are thus set free they move about, interacting with other atoms, and so become responsible for a large proportion of the dose delivered to the irradiated volume. At a particular point of interest, secondary electrons arrive, depositing energy which is included in the computation of absorbed dose. Similarly, other secondary electrons are set into motion at that point and in the surrounding volume, and carry away part of the energy imparted there. When both effects – incoming and outgoing electrons – compensate each other, a situation of so-called electronic equilibrium exists. Electrons come from points upstream in the beam and others move off to points downstream, lying farther ahead (Fig. 2.2).

The position of the maximum in depth-dose curves is explained by the fact that for points in tissue at or near the skin or entrance surface there are far less incoming electrons or none at all, since previous layers of tissue which would serve as a

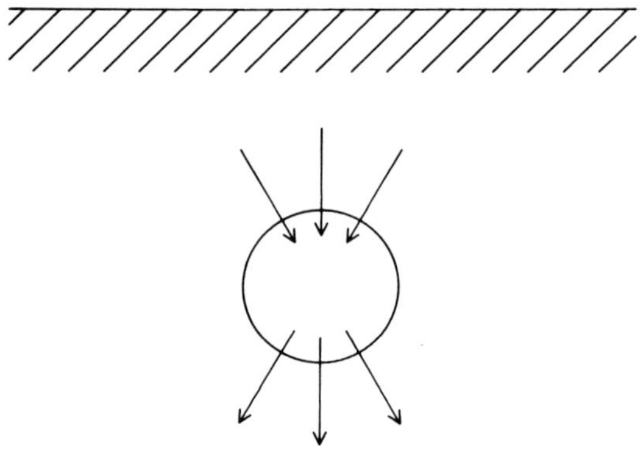

Fig. 2.2. Electronic equilibrium. Energy deposited at a small volume of irradiated material by incoming electrons compensates for energy carried away by outgoing electrons

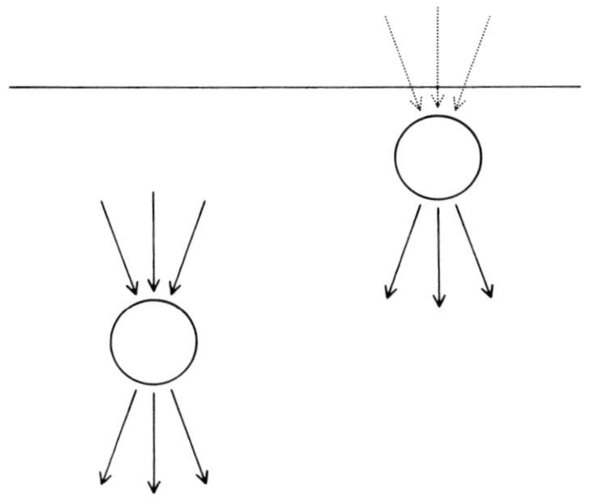

Fig. 2.3. Two distinct situations arise depending on the depth of the volume under consideration from the entrance surface of the exposed medium. On the *left-hand side*, the situation is that of electronic equilibrium. On the *right-hand side*, electronic equilibrium is not attained

source of electrons are lacking; rather there is only air, where the proportion of secondary radiation is negligible (Fig. 2.3).

The lower the beam energy, the closer is the depth of maximum dose to the entrance surface. Since the maximum absorbed dose occurs at the depth at which electronic equilibrium is attained, secondary electrons created in layers of tissue nearer the skin must expend their energy along their tracks and finally come to rest at the point of interest. Electrons will not come to rest at points located before D_{max} – the depth of maximum dose – because their range is higher than that depth. Therefore the value of D_{max} depends on the electron range, which rises as the energy increases (Fig. 2.4).

Only in the case of radiation beams such as diagnostic x-rays, with energies about 10–100 times lower than beams used in radiation therapy, does the maximum dose lie at the entrance surface.

The beam energy is responsible for another two features of electron beam depth-dose curves. First, the slope of the fall-off zone gets steeper as the energy decreases (Fig. 2.5). Second, increasing energy means higher x-ray contamination of the beam. This is represented in Fig. 2.5 as a prolongation of the curves sometimes referred to as a bremsstrahlung tail because it arises when a fraction of the electrons lose their energy through the process of bremsstrahlung, whereby x-rays are produced.

2.2.2 Interaction of Radiation with Matter

The special shapes of the depth-dose curves for x-rays and electrons may be understood on the basis of the different ways these two types of radiation interact with matter at the atomic level. The major difference between x-rays and electrons is that the latter are electrically charged particles and so interact with the electric fields surrounding the nuclei of the elements present in the exposed medium. This interaction is described in terms of an attractive force by Coulomb's law,

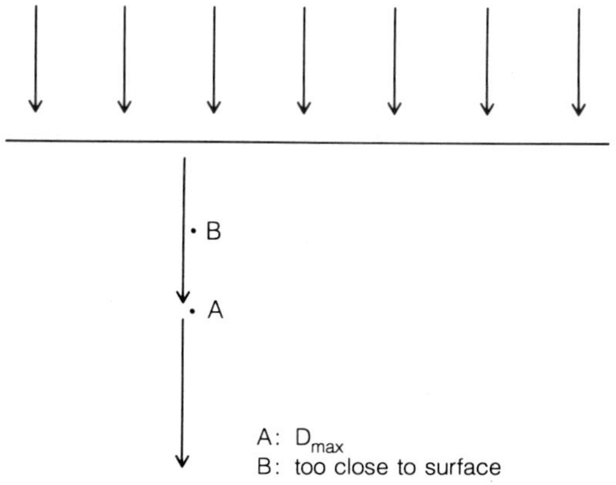

Fig. 2.4. The range of electrons is represented beneath the *horizontal line*. It is seen that no electron can deposit all of its energy at points, such as *point B*, closer to the surface than that range. *Point A*, at the depth of maximum dose, is the point where electronic equilibrum is achieved. Its distance from the surface is equal to the electron range

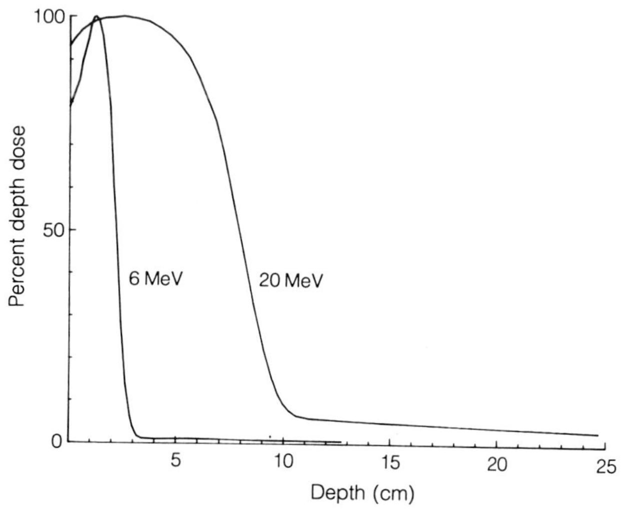

Fig. 2.5. Depth–dose curves for two electron beams of different energies, 6 and 20 MeV

which states that the force attracting the electrons passing by to the nucleus is inversely proportional to the square of the distance between them. This means there is an attraction – low as it may be – even when the electron is still quite distant from the nucleus.

On the other hand, x-rays, which do not have an electric charge, are not subject to this attraction and may travel through matter undisturbed, without giving rise to any interaction until they directly hit one of the electrons bound to an atom of the medium (the collision of x-rays with the nuclei need not be considered since it does not yield any ionization). Therefore, x-rays either collide or they do not: it is a clear-cut question. While electrons may also collide with atomic electrons in the "billiard ball" manner of x-rays, even if they do not the Coulomb interaction is always present.

When collision with atomic electrons occurs, the colliding electron may have sufficient energy to supply the target electron with the amount of energy it needs in order either to break its bonds with the atom and escape from it, the so-called ionization process, or to enter one of the higher energy "excited" states that quantum mechanical rules allow for this atom. These excited states are very unstable and the atom has a natural tendency to return to the previous, more stable lower energy state within a very short time. This is achieved by the electron ridding itself of an amount of energy exactly equal to the energy difference between the two states. This energy is given off by the atom as an x-ray and, since the energy differences between the two states have characteristic values for each element, these x-rays and referred to as characteristic radiation.

When the interaction between electrons and atoms is purely of the Coulomb type, the former travel in a trajectory that bends more and more as they approach the nucleus (Fig. 2.6), very much like a comet passing near the sun. A bending trajectory means a change in velocity, that is, an acceleration. It is well known that accelerated charged particles lose energy by means of electromagnetic radiation. For high energy electrons such as those used in radiotherapy, this radiation consists of x-rays. The process is called radiative collision or "bremsstrahlung."

Because electrons interact all the time, their energy is lost in a continuous way and they come to rest within a very short distance (a few centimeters in tissue) – hence the rapid decline in electron beam depth–dose curves (cf. Fig. 2.1), where the depth equal to the electron range for that energy corresponds to a percentage dose of almost zero.

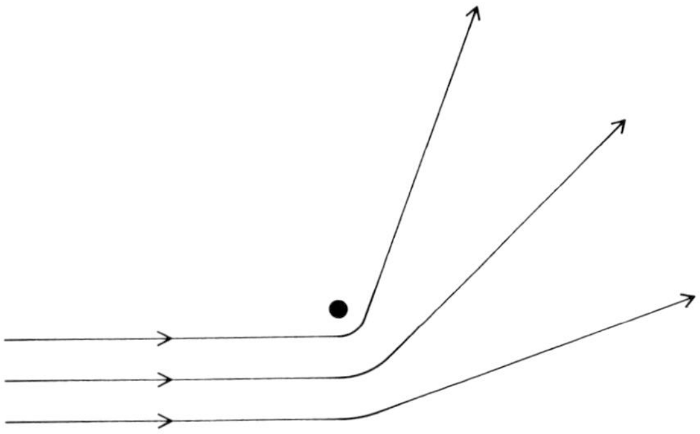

Fig. 2.6. A simplified representation of possible trajectories of electrons passing at different distances from an atomic nucleus, represented by the *circle*

The shape of x-ray depth-dose curves is different due to the above-mentioned fact that a particular x-ray may or may not interact with atomic electrons. Therefore, after the beam has passed through a considerable amount of tissue, a good number of the initial x-rays are still present in it, giving rise to secondary electrons which build up the curve, producing the smooth slope of a decreasing exponential function.

2.2.3 Beam Profiles

In order to know the three-dimensional dose distribution of an electron beam, measurements must be made of absorbed dose in several planes or along various directions. Of special importance are the plots known as beam profiles, consisting of representations of dose versus distance (position) along a straight line usually crossing the beam axis – or central ray – and perpendicular to it, for a particular depth.

For obvious reasons all measurements of dose distribution in tissue are carried out in materials of which the density, atomic number, and other properties are similar to those of human body tissues; such materials are referred to as phantoms.

If a probe is continuously moved inside a water phantom in a direction perpendicular to the beam axis, and the response is recorded on paper by an analog plotter, a curve like that shown in Fig. 2.7 will be obtained. It can be seen that the absorbed dose displays virtually the same values (to within a few percent) at all points inside the beam bound-

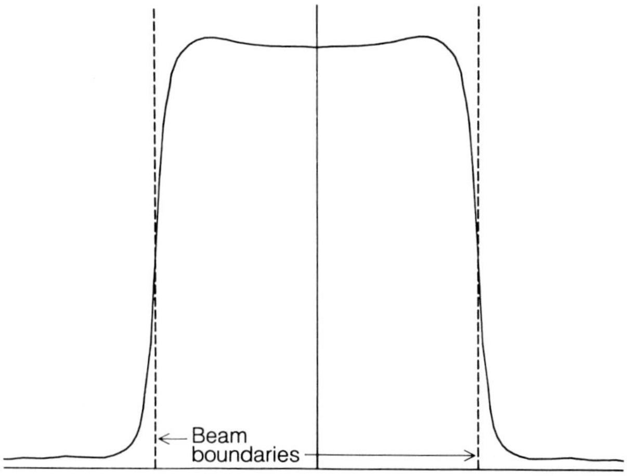

Fig. 2.7. Electron beam dose profile showing relative dose versus distance from the beam axis, represented by the *vertical solid line*

aries except, possibly, for two smooth peaks, one at each side of the profile, called "horns." There is then a rapid decrease in dose at the beam edges, and finally the curve reflects very small values slowly approaching zero outside the beam boundaries. This low dose is known as the peripheral dose, and the narrow zone where the dose has a high gradient building up very rapidly is called the penumbra. Peripheral dose arises due to partial transmission and scatter through the beam-limiting collimators.

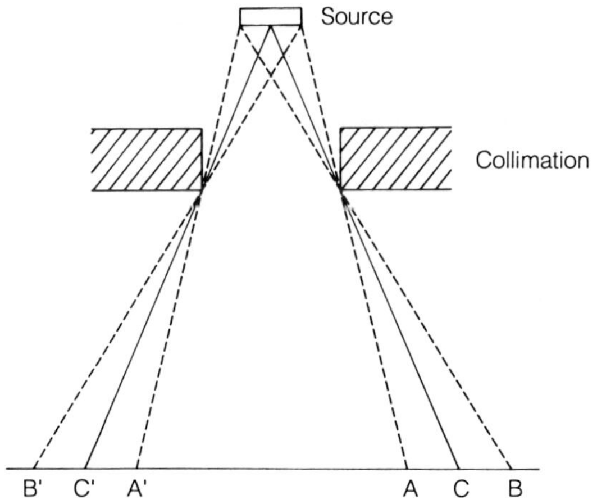

Fig. 2.8. Geometric penumbra. Points lying between *A* and *B* or *A′* and *B′*, such as C or C′, cannot see all the source and therefore receive primary radiation only along those rays not blocked by the collimators. The size of the geometric penumbra depends on the source to collimator distance, on the source to surface distance, and on the size of the source. In the figure, the penumbra is shown exaggeratedly large for illustrative purposes

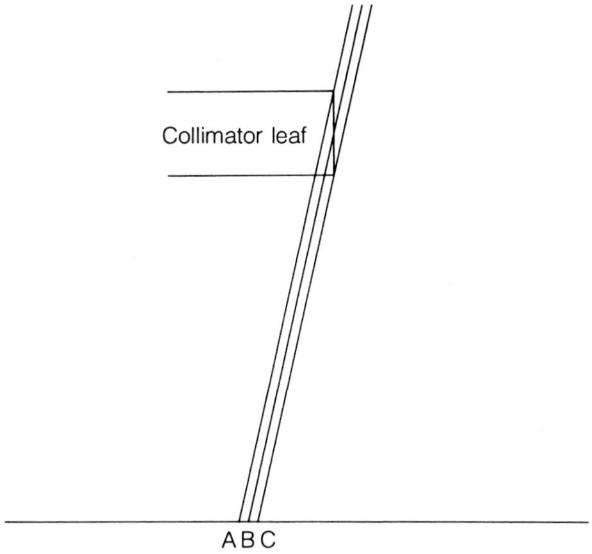

Fig. 2.9. Physical penumbra. Points between *A* and *C*, such as *B*, are partially blocked by the collimator leaf, and consequently receive less radiation than points lying under the direct beam, but more than points completely blocked by the collimators

The penumbra has the same origin as peripheral dose as well as the lack of lateral electronic equilibrium (Johns and Cunningham 1983) and in the fact that the electron beam source is not punctual, i.e., electrons arise not from a point but from a region in space of finite size. In Fig. 2.8, all points between A and A′ see all of the source so they receive all possible radiation. Points lying between A and B or between A′ and B′ can see only part of the source and therefore receive a lower dose. Points beyond B or B′ cannot see the source so they receive only a peripheral dose. The distance between points A and B is a measure of the geometric penumbra, so-called because of the above geometric considerations.

Figure 2.9 illustrates the situation giving rise to the physical penumbra. Different points such as A, B, and C receive radiation which has to pass through different thicknesses of material as determined by the collimator leaf. Thus, the amounts of transmitted radiation will not be the same in every case.

Two important features of an electron beam profile are flatness and symmetry. Flatness means homogeneity, i.e., that all points in the useful region of the beam will receive a uniform dose. Of course, in practice the requirement is that dose differences between two points are less than

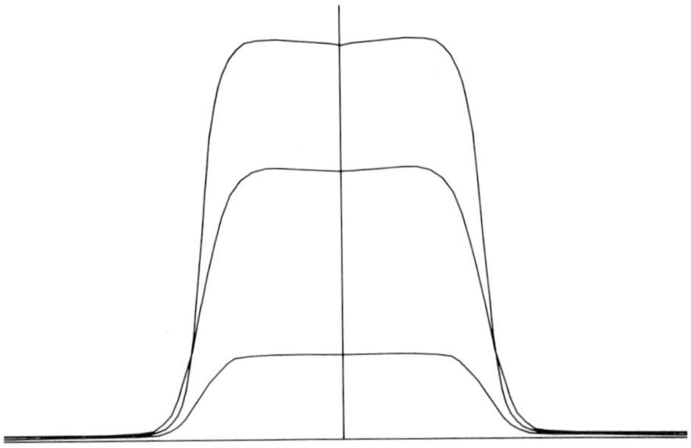

Fig. 2.10. Electron beam profiles at various depths

a given reasonable value, since perfect flatness is impossible to achieve.

Flatness will depend on the depth at which the profile has been obtained. In Fig. 2.10 different profiles can be seen for an electron beam at various depths.

Flatness is an obvious requirement if the treated area of the body is to receive a uniform dose. Symmetry is also important for this reason, and for those depths where the profile is no longer flat, symmetry grants a uniform dose to points lying at the same distance from the beam axis.

In linear accelerators, flatness and symmetry are monitored by various means, such as focusing coils and quadrupole magnets which steer the beam in the right direction, or flattening foils, made out of low atomic number materials, that absorb the electron beam in a nonuniform way so as to flatten out a beam originally having the shape of a gaussian or narrower peak.

2.2.4 Isodose Curves

A different way to visualize a three-dimensional dose distribution, instead of plotting dose versus position along a line, consists in representing a set of closed curves connecting all points having the same absorbed dose value.

Fig. 2.11. Isodose curves for a photon beam (*left*) and an electron beam (*right*)

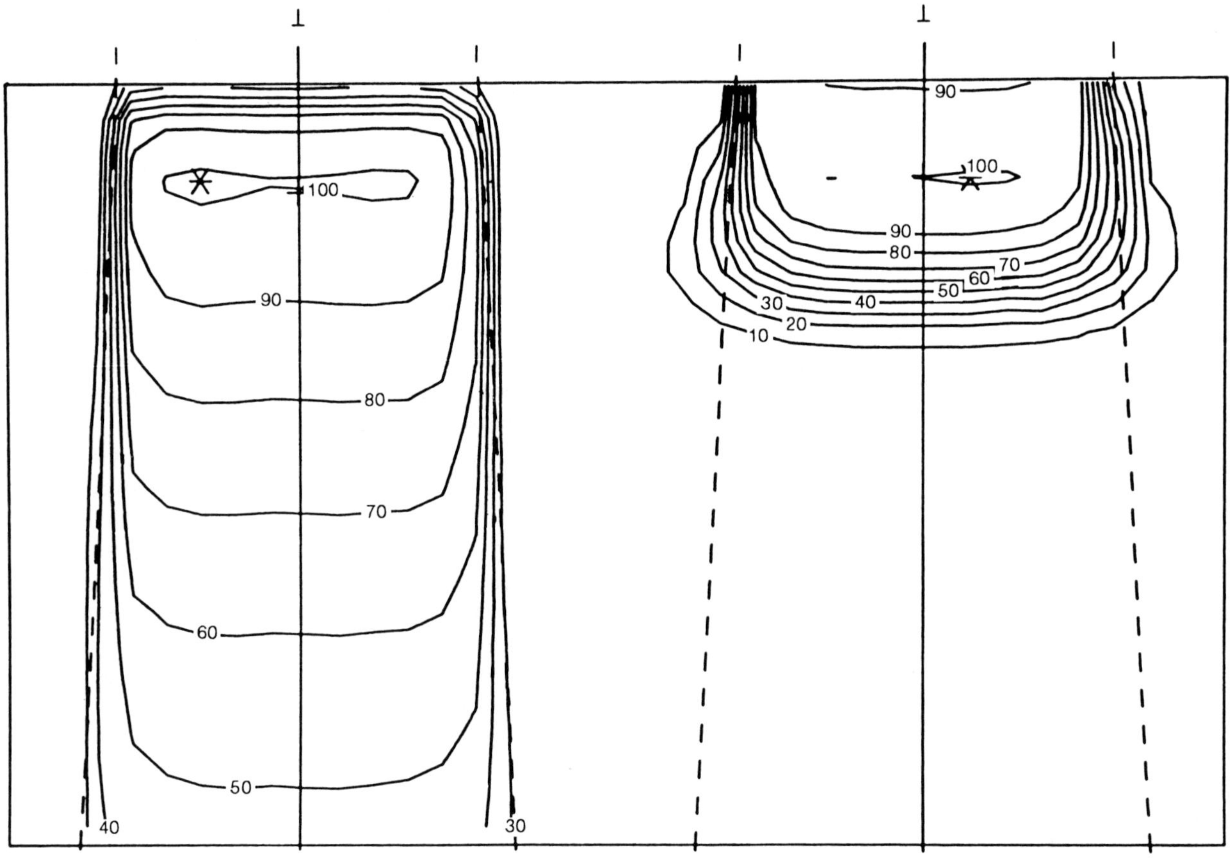

In a three-dimensional picture, one would deal with isodose surfaces but a more straightforward view of the distribution is obtained if these surfaces are cut by planes. These planes are usually parallel or perpendicular to the central axis of the beam, and the intersections between them and the isodose surfaces form the isodose curves.

If a set of isodose curves is measured for a particular beam and is then utilized in a particular patient who is to undergo radiation therapy, it is possible to see at first glance how the dose will be distributed inside the patient's body. The advantage of having sets of isodose charts is thus obvious.

Nonetheless, a patient's body does not have a flat surface and the inner density is not uniform but heterogeneous. For these reasons, the measured isodose curves need to be corrected since they are usually obtained in water phantoms. These corrections are always cumbersome to apply but do not represent a serious drawback when performed with the aid of a computer.

In Fig. 2.11, isodose curves for photons and electrons are shown: the dramatic difference in penetration of these types of radiation can be envisaged. Both sets of curves correspond to measurements performed in a water phantom. Figure 2.12 illustrates the result of application of a set of isodose curves for an electron beam to a cross-sectional contour, after all the necessary corrections have been applied.

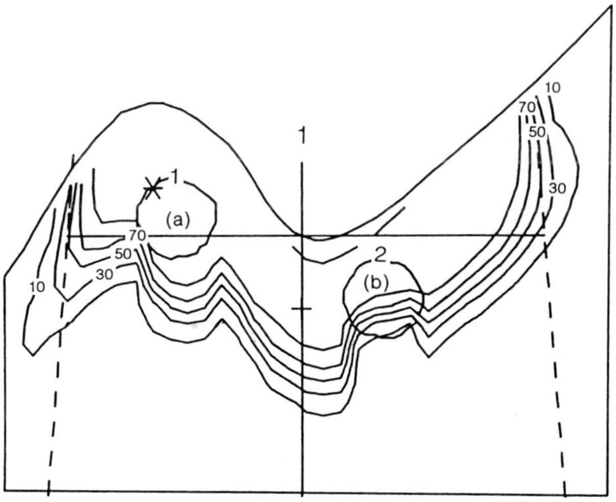

Fig. 2.12. Isodose curves for an electron beam irradiating a medium limited by a curved (nonflat) surface and having regions of low density (*a*) and high density (*b*). Region (*a*) lets more radiation through, whereas region (*b*) absorbs more radiation

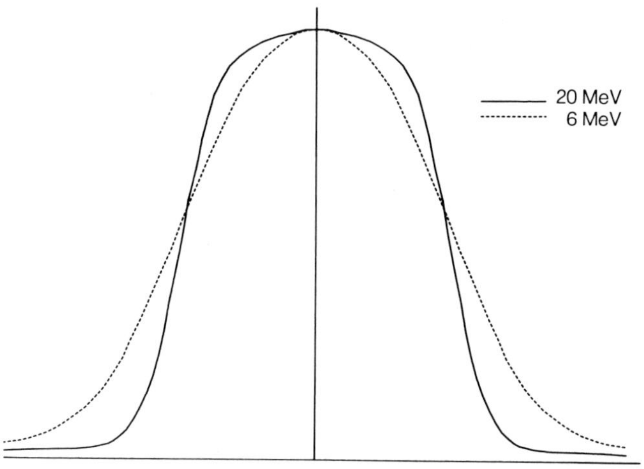

Fig. 2.13. Electron beam dose profiles after the beam has passed through the primary collimating system

2.3 Description of Applicators for External Beam Radiotherapy

As it leaves the accelerator head the electron beam does not yet have its ultimate shape. After the beam has passed through a flattening foil, the dose profile still looks far from flat, as Fig. 2.13 shows for two different beam energies.

In order to flatten the profile further and to reduce the penumbra to an acceptable minimum, devices known as applicators are mounted on the accelerator head. Figure 2.14 shows one such applicator. Its upper part consists of a thin plate made out of aluminum, which serves as a secondary collimator after the beam has passed through the x-ray jaws and reduces the peripheral dose. This is the part that is attached to the machine head and is sometimes referred to as the mounting plate.

Electrons traveling down the beam first pass through the opening on the upper slab and then continue on their way to the patient's skin. A fraction of them are scattered at the walls of the aluminum cone and are used to fill up the beam. This fraction, though, can be as much as 40% of the tumor dose (McCullough and Anderson 1982). As they are mainly of low energy, the dose to the skin would be considerably increased were it not for the aluminum trimmers at the lower part of the applicator, which are kept in contact with the patient's skin. These are used to produce a sharper penumbra and to ensure that no more than 1% of the dose at the treatment field comes from electrons scattered at the walls of the cone.

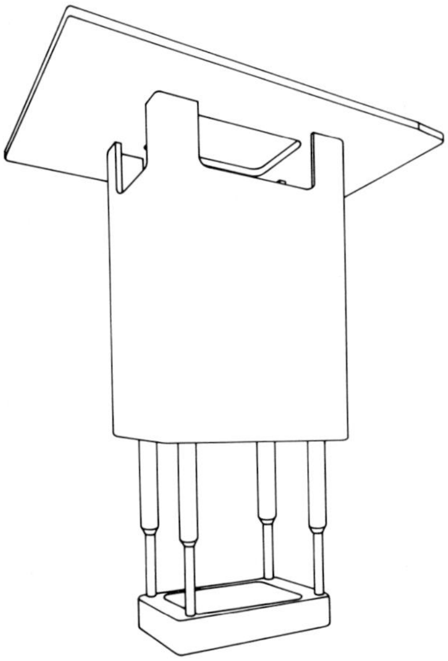

Fig. 2.14. Applicator for external beam radiotherapy manufactured by Siemens

Other methods employed for homogenizing the dose include separate trimming leaves to be mounted on the x-ray jaws so as to allow any rectangular field size within the permitted range, instead of having a set of several fixed size applicators.

It is obvious that these devices are not practical for IORT because good dose distributions require the lower trimming part to be in contact with the treated structure or tumor. In IORT, this portion should be introduced inside the surgical incision during treatment, and this is not always feasible.

Moreover, the patient is normally treated on the operating table itself, and one may not always have complete freedom to move it up and down so as to bring the patient into contact with the applicator. Finally, the design and manufacture of applicators specifically suited for IORT often incorporate new features which optimize them for the task in question, but which would be of little or no interest in external beam radiotherapy. This is the case, for example, with the viewing system, which has no rationale in conventional external radiotherapy but which helps one to aim the beam accurately toward the target in IORT. Consequently, it is clear that the design, manufacture, and calibration of a new, special type of applicator are among the priorities of an IORT program.

2.4 Applicators for IORT as Designed at the Clinica Universitaria de Navarra

Almost all institutions involved in IORT programs have developed their own sets of applicators and, aside from the optimizing details, the basic layout is similar in almost every case.

A plastic tube usually having a circular, rectangular, or "squircle" (Fraass et al. 1985) cross-section is able to slide up and down a metallic applicator or a docking adapter which is inserted in the accelerator head.

The original applicator designed at the Clinica Universitaria de Navarra (C.U.N.) is depicted in Fig. 2.15, along with the corresponding 3 mm thick cylindrical methacrylate tube, which docks directly into the upper aluminum structure. The tube is clamped at a particular position by means of an aluminum ring that may be easily hand-held and rotated around the cone so as to squeeze a silicone ring around the tube to prevent it from sliding downward.

This simple design makes these applicators extremely easy and straightforward to handle. Gas sterilization of both plastic tubes and metallic cones is also facilitated. On the other hand, with this arrangement the entire applicator and not just

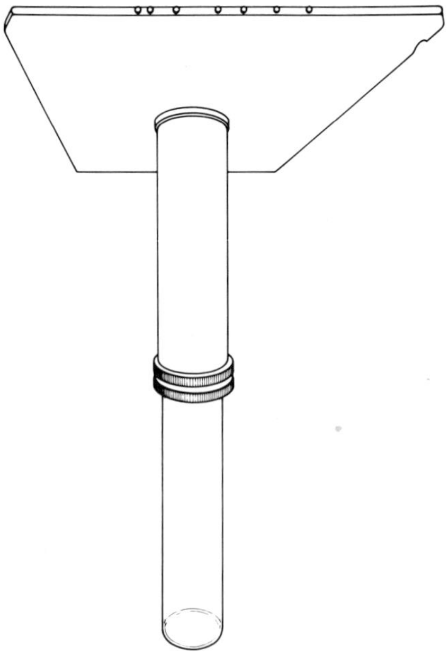

Fig. 2.15. Applicator for IORT designed and manufactured by the Clinica Universitaria de Navarra

the tube must be substituted if the cross-sectional size of the tube does not fit the area to be treated. This clearly constitutes a disadvantage and other types of applicator are preferable which enable the normally heavy metallic part to be left mounted during the whole procedure without need of further tampering with it. Such applicators are usually more complicated because they consist of several metallic parts to allow correct docking of plastic tubes of various sizes (FRAASS et al. 1985). Sometimes, the tubes themselves are built with one end adapted for docking into a unique cone (MCCULLOUGH and ANDERSON 1982), without any need for an adapting intermediate part. Both methods allow quick attachment or removal of different plastic tubes without having to move the rest of the applicator.

The aluminum cone of these applicators serves the purpose of scattering electrons off its walls for building up the electron field. The plastic tube is transparent to allow vision through it, and permits physical separation of normal anatomic structures at risk from structures to be included in the treatment field.

Plastic tubes of circular cross-section are most often employed (MCCULLOUGH and GUNDERSON 1988). For each diameter, several tubes exist, with one end cut at different bevel angles. This is very useful in many situations in which it is not possible for technical reasons to set up the applicator so that the plastic tube is perpendicular to the tumor bed or the surface to be exposed to the radiation beam.

The IORT applicators manufactured at the C.U.N. are tubes with bevel angles of 15°, 30°, and 45°, which about cover all practical needs. Each tube has both ends differently beveled, including 0° (no bevel) and can be used with either end toward the tumor.

Whenever it is not possible to set up a standard source-to-tumor distance because of restrictions in moving the operating table, the tube may be slid up or down by the required amount so that its lower end is in contact with the tumor or tumor bed. The new treatment distance is then read off from a meter scale alongside the tube on which positive and negative offsets from a standard distance are indicated. Another scale lies reversed (upside down) on the opposite side of the tube, for those cases in which the other end of the tube is the one in contact with the tumor, depending on which bevel angle is chosen.

2.5 Dosimetry of IORT Applicators

2.5.1 Introduction

The fact that special applicators for IORT are designed with shapes different from those of standard applicators introduces geometric factors that have an influence over dose distributions. This influence has turned out to be more quantitative than qualitative in the sense that the new dose distributions look very much like those in conventional treatment.

Parameters used to characterize the dose distribution have new values usually differing from the previous ones by only small amounts. In a few extreme cases these differences grow far too large and may yield unwanted inhomogeneities in dose distributions. For this reason, minor modifications to the IORT applicators are being sought in order to improve those distributions which have become unacceptable.

Not all the changes found in the new distributions have been for the worse. On the contrary, a few parameters have been so changed that their new values turn out to be highly desirable. It is often found, however, that modifications which result in the improvement of a certain parameter produce worse values in respect of another. This leads in most cases to trade-offs in order to reach compromises. These trade-offs mostly involve the treatment settings, such as the x-ray jaw opening and the treatment distance.

Calibration of IORT applicators includes studies of dose distribution by means of depth–dose data, beam profiles, and isodose curves. Also of importance are output factors and distance correction factors.

For beam profiles, penumbra, peripheral dose, flatness, and symmetry must be considered. Depth–dose parameters of relevance are:

- Surface dose
- Depth of 90% dose
- Slope of fall-off portion of the depth–dose curve
- Practical range
- x-ray contamination by bremsstrahlung

2.5.2 Output Factors

For practical reasons, among which the most important are the limited range of vertical movement of the operating table and the original length of the plastic tubes as supplied by the manufacturer, the standard source-to-tumor distance for IORT with the C.U.N.-made applicators is greater than that for external beam radiotherapy, namely 116 cm instead of 100 cm. Therefore, it was important to check whether dose rate had diminished and, if so, to what extent. Prescribed doses in IORT protocols are in the range of 10–20 Gy at the C.U.N. It is important to have a relatively high dose rate to avoid procedures of long duration. It was found that dose rates for applicators with tubes of different diameters and for different energies had values ranging from 35% lower up to 20% higher as compared with dose rates for a standard (Siemens) 15 × 15 cm square applicator for external beam radiotherapy.

The treatment times have not been substantially different from those with conventional applicators and source-to-tumor distances in external irradiation; they have generally ranged from 2 to 8 min, although in a few cases there have been higher values of up to 20 min. These were extreme situations in which very high prescribed doses were combined with long treatment distances and tube diameters and energies for which the output was lowest.

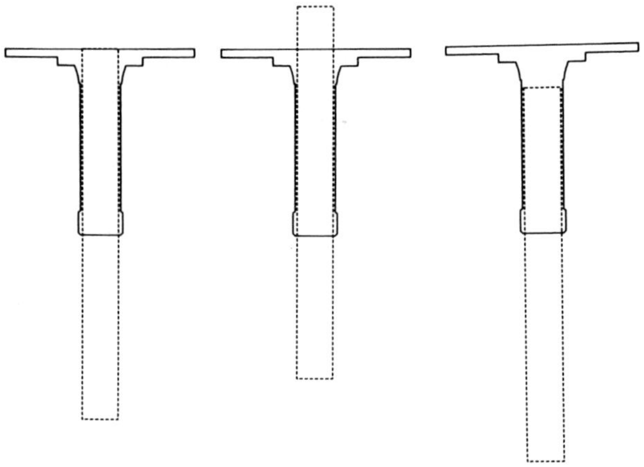

Fig. 2.16. Representation of the relative position of the plastic tube (*dashed lines*) with respect to the applicator for standard treatment distance (*left*) and other treatment distances (*center and right*)

2.5.3 Distance Correction Factors

Since the inverse square law does not generally hold for electron beams, measurements were carried out of dose rate for every diameter and energy at the depth of maximum dose, over a span of distances ranging from 95 cm through 138 cm, although most of the time treatment distances differed from the standard one of 116 cm by no more than 2 cm.

The standard treatment distance of 116 cm occurs when the lower end of the tube is in contact with the tumor and the upper end is at the same level as the upper surface of the applicator mount.

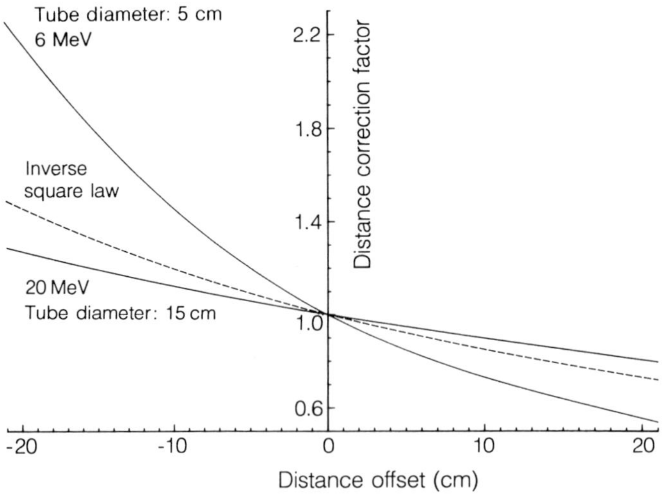

Fig. 2.17. A distance correction factor is plotted against distance offset from the standard treatment distance for the two cones for which deviation from the inverse square law is maximum: the tube diameter of 5 cm and energy of 6 MeV, and the tube diameter of 15 cm and energy of 20 MeV. All other cones show an intermediate behavior. A plot of the inverse square law is included for comparison

Other distances arise when the tube must be held farther up or down than the previous position (Fig. 2.16). Figure 2.17 shows some of the results. A distance correction factor, defined as the ratio of dose rate at actual treatment distance to dose rate at standard distance, is plotted versus the difference between these distances for two extreme cases. Inverse square law correction factors are included for comparison. It can be seen that deviations from the inverse square law can be relatively large. The largest deviations occur for low energies and small tube diameters.

It can be seen that between the case of low energies and small diameters and the case of high energies and large diameters there will be some cases for which deviation from the inverse square law will be minimal.

2.5.4 Depth–Dose Data

2.5.4.1 Surface Dose (Entrance Dose)

The absorbed dose at the entrance point, which is the skin in conventional treatment, is relatively high for electron beams. Since in IORT the tumor or tumor bed is under direct exposure with no layers of healthy tissue having to be traversed by radiation, it will play the role of the skin and will receive a relatively high dose. The higher the beam energy, the higher the surface dose will be.

For those cases of low beam energies such that the entrance dose is sensibly lower than 90%, the usual reference isodose for dose prescription, bolus is used to improve homogeneity over the target volume, which includes an increase in surface dose.

Surface dose values for the C.U.N.-manufactured IORT applicators present values sensibly a few percent higher than the corresponding values for the Siemens external beam applicators. Of course, this is highly desirable since it contributes to a more homogeneous tumor dose.

2.5.4.2 Depth of Maximum Dose

A slight difference between the two types of applicator under comparison is found when the depth of maximum dose is considered. This depth is shifted a few millimeters toward the entrance surface in the case of IORT applicators. This would be expected to limit the tumors that can be treated, in accordance with their thickness in the beam direction. In practice, however, most IORT procedures deal with partially or totally resected tumors and this makes the low energies the usual choice for treatment.

The reason why surface dose is increased and the depth of maximum dose reduced in IORT applicators is again the extra amount of electrons scattered from the plastic tube, which build up the dose at the beam entrance layers.

2.5.5 Beam Profiles

Beam profiles for electron beams with almost any applicator designed for IORT show the so-called horns or hot spots, that is, a relatively large increase in dose at the beam boundaries. This is due to scattering of electrons off the plastic tube which extends all the way down to the tumor or tumor bed.

A typical beam profile is shown in Fig. 2.18. The higher the energy, the more pronounced are the horns. Also, horns are more liable to occur for large tube diameters because in small diameter tubes they tend to be compensated by the fact that the penumbra begins very near the beam's central axis.

Horn heterogeneity may be as great as 10%–15% at the depth of maximum dose, and even more than that (20%) for points lying nearer the entrance surface. This is the worst situation, in which very large tube diameters and high energies are used.

The horn effect builds up the beam at its edges and this has the consequence of sharpening it, and therefore of reducing the penumbra.

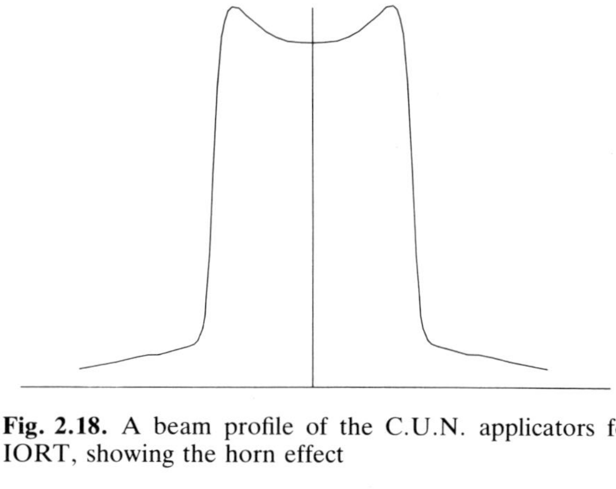

Fig. 2.18. A beam profile of the C.U.N. applicators for IORT, showing the horn effect

Aside from the heterogeneity introduced by the horns, beam profiles are symmetric, as would be expected, since the IORT applicators are themselves symmetric with respect to the beam central axis.

Another unwanted effect which may arise, depending on the applicator design, is an increase in dose in areas out of but near the tube, known as peripheral dose, as mentioned earlier. This increase is also due to scatter at the tube walls and, unlike with standard applicators for external beam radiotherapy, there are no aluminum trimmers to reduce it. Peripheral dose in the C.U.N.-manufactured IORT applicators is important only for depths between zero (entrance surface) and the depth of maximum dose. It also increases with beam energy and tube diameter, and for the worst cases it may amount to 15%.

2.6 Results

From the clinical point of view, the two major inconveniences of the above-described applicators for IORT are the high peripheral dose and the hot spots, or horns, near the beam boundaries.

Peripheral dose can be partially reduced by choosing a suitably small x-ray jaw opening. This is not always feasible or convenient in actual practice, since it means having different openings and, consequently, different applicator coding for each tube diameter. If the x-ray jaw opening chosen is too small, the penumbra might be influenced and perhaps increased as well. The easiest way to reduce peripheral dose to acceptable amounts consists in employing a suitable material as part of the mounting plate or attached to it, to increase the electron absorption. Choice materials are lead and brass, the latter being preferable due to its lower bremsstrahlung x-ray production compared with lead (Palta and Suntharalingam 1989).

As for the horns that arise by the streaming of electrons scattered at the plastic walls of the tube, a very straightforward method to correct them is the inclusion of a plastic or metal ring around the tube. This ring intercepts most of the scattered electrons that cause the horns. If the ring is made out of a suitable metal, the electrons are also spread out at large angles (Palta and Suntharalingam 1989), with the result of additional beam uniformity. Suitable metals include steel, brass, and copper.

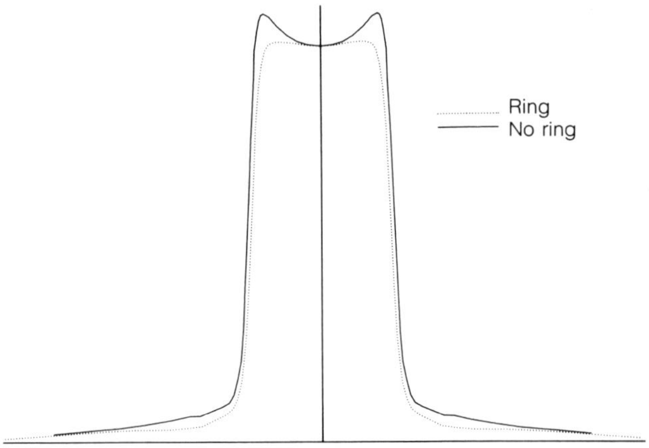

Fig. 2.19. Correction of horns by means of the insertion of a brass ring around the plastic tube

At the C.U.N., brass rings have been tested with several combinations of thickness and inner diameter, the outer diameter being the same as the inner diameter of the tube. Inner diameters of 1.5 and 3 mm gave good and very similar results, while a thickness of 7 mm was sufficient for the purpose. Later this thickness was increased to 20 mm in order to include a few notches on the ring where a bottom section of the tube could be easily attached or removed so as to have different bevel angles. This had no noticeable effect on the dosimetric results.

The important parameter upon which the "horn" effect was found to be dramatically dependent was the position of the ring, and its distance from the lower edge of the tube. It was found that good results were obtained for a ring position of about 10 cm from the bottom end of the tube. In Fig. 2.19 the difference can be seen between beam profiles obtained with and without a metal ring. Additionally, it can be observed that the beam's effective diameter is slightly reduced due to the fact that the ring's inner diameter is less than that of the plastic tube.

References

Beck C (1907) Über Kombinationsbehandlung bei bösartigen Neubildungen. Berl Klin Wochenschr 44: 1335

Beck C (1909) On external roentgen of internal structures (eventration treatment). NY Med J 89: 621

Fraass BA, Miller RW, Kinsella TJ et al. (1985) Intraoperative radiation therapy at the National Cancer Institute: technical innovations and dosimetry. Int J Radiat Oncol Biol Phys 11: 1299–1311

Johns HE, Cunningham JR (1983) The physics of radiology. Charles C. Thomas, Springfield, Ill

McCullough EC, Anderson JA (1982) The dosimetric properties of an applicator system for intraoperative electron-beam therapy utilizing a clinac-18 accelerator. Med Phys: 261–268

McCullough EC, Gunderson LL (1988) Energy as well as applicator size and shape utilized in over 200 intraoperative electron beam procedures. Int J Radiat Oncol Biol Phys 15: 1041–1042

Mevatron 77 Instruction Manual, Siemens Medical Laboratories, Inc

Palta JR, Suntharalingam N (1989) A non-docking intraoperative electron beam applicator system. Int J Radiat Oncol Biol Phys 17: 411–417

3 Anesthesia and Hospital Coordination

DAVID ORTIZ DE URBINA, ENRICO TANGCO, JOSÉ LUIS ARROYO, and FRANCISCO CARRASCOSA

CONTENTS

3.1 Introduction 25
3.2 Patients, Methods, and Materials 25
3.2.1 Patient Characteristics 25
3.2.2 Personnel Needed in IORT 26
3.2.3 Anesthetic Considerations 26
3.2.4 Preoperative Evaluation 26
3.2.5 Preanesthetic Medication 26
3.2.6 Patient Transport 27
3.2.7 Post-IORT Evaluation 30
3.3 Complications 30
References 30

3.1 Introduction

Intraoperative radiotherapy is a treatment modality designed to combine the efforts of surgery and radiotherapy to increase local tumor control rates in cancer therapy. The possibility of treating during cancer surgery different areas with electron beams, delivering high single doses of radiation, while normal uninvolved tissues are mobilized or protected, has been attractive to both surgeons and radiotherapists. Other advantages of IORT are better delineation of the area involved by tumor and a reduction in tumor burden by surgical resection. Several aspects of this modality are of particular interest to anesthesiologists (FRIESEN et al. 1987):

- The anesthetic procedure involves a high risk because of the patients' poor physical status, which is caused by both their disease and previous treatment modalities such as surgery, external beam radiotherapy, and chemotherapy.
- Major tumor resections involve very aggressive surgery of long duration.
- It is necessary to perform the surgery in the operating room, then to transport the anesthetized patient, with an open surgical wound (not exposed), through halls, elevators, and public spaces to reach and return from the linear accelerator room.
- The anesthetized patient is treated in a linear accelerator while all attendant personnel are away from the immediate vicinity of the patient during irradiation.
- Radiation treatment adds approximately 60 min to the anesthetic time, of which 45 min are spent outside the operating room.

In this chapter we shall discuss the anesthetic management of patients undergoing IORT by reference to the protocol designed at the Clinica Universitaria de Navarra (C.U.N.). The Department of Anesthesiology is responsible for preoperative evaluation, anesthetic support, and ensuring that vital signs are stable during perioperative and postoperative periods.

3.2 Patients, Methods, and Materials

3.2.1 Patient Characteristics

Between September 1984 and June 1989, 468 patients (296 males and 172 females) underwent IORT at the C.U.N. The mean age of the group was 43 years (range: 2–80 years). All types of tumor histology have been included in this study, and Table 3.1 shows the frequency of surgery in different anatomic locations.

The mean duration of surgery was 4 h (range: 2–12 h). The mean duration of exposure to radiation was 6 min (range: 2.5–20 min), the time in each case depending on the number of IORT fields treated and the characteristics of the procedure (cone diameter, electron energy, dose, and source–target distance).

DAVID ORTIZ DE URBINA, Dr., ENRICO TANGCO, Dr., Radiotherapy Division, Department of Oncology, JOSÉ L. ARROYO, Dr., FRANCISCO CARRASCOSA, Dr., Consultant, Department of Anesthesiology, Clinica Universitaria de Navarra, 31080 Pamplona, Spain

Table 3.1. Types of surgery performed during the initial 5 years' experience with IORT

Type of surgery	No. of patients	%
Neurosurgery	13	2
Head and neck	15	3
Thoracic	69	14
Abdominal (gastrointestinal)	139	29
Gynecologic	26	5
Urologic	53	11
Orthopedic	121	25
Other	32	6
Total	468	100

3.2.2 Personnel Needed in IORT

The development of IORT techniques requires close cooperation among surgeons, anesthesiologists, and radiotherapists, as well as a suitable support team of specialist nurses well versed in radiotherapy techniques and surgical instrumentation. On average 11 people are needed for every procedure (Table 3.2).

3.2.3 Anesthetic Considerations

It has been reported that IORT presents the anesthesiologist with various challenges (Bashein et al. 1986; Hodel and Martin 1989). Correct amnesia and analgesia must be achieved, as must inhibition of sensory and autonomic reflexes and complete skeletal muscle relaxation. General anesthesia is the procedure of choice because it achieves all these objectives. The unavailability of a single anesthetic agent able to produce an adequate deeper level of anesthesia with a wide margin of security for toxicity means there is a need to combine several drugs (neuroleptanesthesia).

3.2.4 Preoperative Evaluation

A preanesthetic anamnesis and a complete physical examination are two essential aspects of the preoperative evaluation of the patient. The physical examination is performed the day before surgery, and special attention is paid to weight, height, body surface area, and cardiopulmonary and neurologic status. A history of previous surgery is also important.

Table 3.2. Personnel needed in IORT

1 or 2 surgeons
1 or 2 anesthesiologists
2 radiation oncologists
1 physicist
2 radiotherapy nurses and/or technicans
2 surgical nurses

Factors that make anesthesia a high risk procedure are as follows:

- Age greater than 65 years
- Karnofsky performance status of less than 70%
- Nutritional and/or hydration problems
- Prior treatment with hepatotoxic, cardiotoxic, nephrotoxic, or pulmonary toxic drugs
- Prior treatment with drugs causing myelosuppression
- Drug interactions with anesthetics
- Prior cardiopulmonary disease
- External beam radiotherapy (radical doses) of large areas, with vital organs included in the radiation field.

Important tests in the preoperative evaluation of IORT patients are listed in Table 3.3

3.2.5 Preanesthetic Medication

Drugs are administered in accordance with the patient's age sex, weight, physical and mental status, and the type of surgery to be performed. Initially, the objectives are to obtain sedation, amnesia, and analgesia, and elimination of invol-

Table 3.3. Preoperative evaluation of IORT patients

Hemoglobin, hematocrit, platelets
Coagulation
Bleeding time
Coagulation time
Prothrombin time
Partial thromboplastin time
Blood and Rh group
Biochemical levels (electrolytes, creatinine, glucose, urea)
Hepatic function test
Renal function test
Respiratory function test[a]
ECG monitoring
Cardiologic studies (echocardiography, stress testing)[b]

[a] Patients with chronic obstructive or restrictive pulmonary disease
[b] Patients with previous cardiac disease and/or patients over 65

untary reflexes and nausea and vomiting. In our protocol bromazepam and atropine are used.

Prior to the induction of anesthesia, the following procedures are performed:

- Insertion of two large-bore peripheral intravenous cannulas and another central line (internal jugular or subclavian vein)
- Insertion of a catheter in the femoral or radial artery
- Monitoring of direct arterial and central venous pressure
- Monitoring of urinary output
- ECG monitoring

In the operating room the selection of anesthetic agents and techniques depends on both the patient's preoperative status and the planned surgical procedure.

3.2.5.1 Drugs Used in Induction of Anesthesia

Anesthetic induction is achieved with either intravenous barbiturates or inhalation anesthetics. We generally use a combination of thiopental (an ultrashort acting barbiturate), fentanyl (a narcotic analgesic), pancuronium (a non-depolarizing neuromuscular blocking agent), and benzodiazepines/etomidate.

3.2.5.2 Drugs Used in Maintenance of Anesthesia

After the induction of the anesthesia and intubation, anesthesia is maintained with a combination of enflurane (30%) (a volatile anesthetic), nitrous oxide (N_2O: 50%), fentanyl, and pancuronium.

A Draeger model respirator and an Anemone monitor are used. Information is supplied about the tidal volume, the minute volume, the respiratory rate, maximum pressure, positive end-expiratory pressure, inspired oxygen concentration (FiO_2), and temperature.

There is an alarm device to draw attention to undesirable changes in ventilatory pattern: minute volume (0–40 liters/min), instantaneous pressure (0–99 mbar), and FiO_2 (18%–99% molO_2).

During the replacement and maintenance of volume support, the following drugs are used:

- Crystalloids: 0.9% sodium chloride, 0.33% NaCl dextrose, $NaHCO_3$ 1/6 M
- Colloids: dextran 70, human albumin
- Red cell concentrate and/or whole blood (if there is massive hemorrhage).

Preoperative monitoring includes several other parameters besides standard analytical blood determinations (hemoglobin, hematocrit, total proteins, electrolytes, acid-base balance).

3.2.6 Patient Transport

3.2.6.1 Transportation System

The transportation system used at C.U.N. consists of:

- A transporting carriage–operating table unit
- A unit for the transportation of accessory material

The transporting carriage–operating table unit consists of:

- A transporting chassis
- An operating table
- Chassis motion control systems
- Locking systems

For patient transportation we use a chassis supported on wheels (Fig. 3.1) which has a perfect docking system for clamping to the operating table. This system ensures simplicity of transporta-

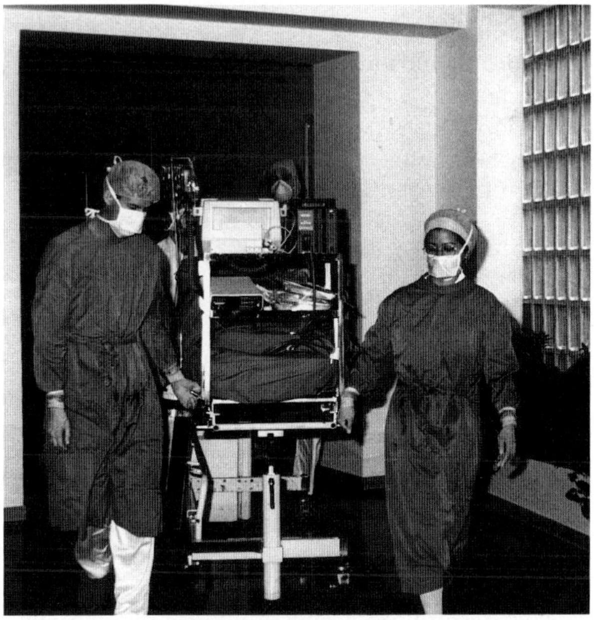

Fig. 3.1. Transportation procedure: general view

tion from the operating room to the radiotherapy facilities and back to the operating room since it is secure and also ensures that there is no need to move the patient from one table to another.

There are four motion possibilities to allow any setup which the radiotherapist or anesthesiologist may require (up–down, anterior–posterior, right–lateral, left–lateral, and Trendelenberg), as well as a locking system for the whole unit.

The unit for transportation of accessory material consists of (a) a trolley for transportation of monitoring devices, resuscitation equipment, and medication, and (b) a clamping device for the oxygen tank. The portable cart couples to the rear portion of the operating table through a lateral locking system. The oxygen tank is clamped by means of two stainless steel hooks to one side, lateral with respect to the major axis of the operating table; this assures good ventilation of the patient during transport, avoiding risks such as accidental disconnection of the oxygen tank.

3.2.6.2 Operating Room – Radiotherapy Unit – Operating Room

In our institution the patient must be moved from the operating room to the radiation unit and back again, through an elevator and some 200 meters of corridors (half of which are through the outpatient section). The safety of patient transport requires that the following be achieved in the operating room:

- Surgical hemostasis
- Adequate blood and hydroelectrolytic replacement
- Cardiovascular stability
- Good oxygenation of the patient

Immediately after these conditions have been established, sterile gauze is placed over the surgical field, after which a small sterile drape is placed. A thin sheet of adherent plastic (steri-drape) is then placed to cover the surgical field. After this, two layers of large sterile drapes are placed to cover the patient before transport begins.

After the transporting chassis has been coupled to the operating table (without transferring the patient from table to table), we make use of the portable monitoring devices (Table 3.4) and assisted respiration is substituted by manual ventilation (ambu-bag).

Table 3.4. Monitoring of IORT patients at different stages of treatment

Operating room	During transport	During IORT
ECG monitoring	ECG monitoring	ECG monitoring
Arterial blood pressure	Arterial blood pressure	Arterial blood pressure
Central venous pressure	Pulse oximetry	Spirometry
Urinary output		
Temperature		
Muscle relaxation		
Spirometry		
FiO_2		
Airways pressure		
Pulse oximetry		
Capnography		

The Critikon Dinamap (Monitor 8100) monitor can display the ECG and numerical data on arterial pressure (systolic, diastolic, and mean arterial pressure), heart rate, and temperature. A pulse oximeter (Ohmeda Biox 3740) measures hemoglobin oxygen saturation.

During transportation, the patient is ventilated with 100% O_2, and anesthesia is maintained with intravenous agents. To ensure the amnesia and hypnosis of the patient, benzodiazepine is used. Besides this, to ensure skeletal muscle relaxation, complete patient immobilization, and correct normal ventilation, a supplementary dose of a nondepolarizing neuromuscular blocking agent (pancuronium) is administered.

The average transportation time between the operating room and the radiation therapy facilities is about 6 min. The cardiopulmonary resuscitation equipment is conveyed with the transporting unit (Table 3.5).

3.2.6.3 Considerations Before IORT

At the radiotherapy unit, several steps need to be taken before IORT:

- Ensure adequate ventilation of the patient:
  a) Check the proper positioning of the endotracheal tube.
  b) Aspirate secretions.
  c) Substitute manual ventilation by mechanical ventilation: the patient is reconnected to the central oxygen supply and volatile anesthetic agents.

Table 3.5. Equipment and drugs used for support of IORT patients

Equipment	Drugs	Others
Laryngoscope	Epinephrine	0.9% NaCl
Endotracheal tubes	Lidocaine	$NaHCO_3$ 1 M
Mask	Methoxamine	10% Macrodex
Ambu bag	Ephedrine	Human albumin
Oxygen tank	Atropine	Packet RBC (2)
Stethoscope	$NaHCO_3$	
ECG monitor	Calcium chloride	
Defibrillator	Corticosteroids	
Sphygmomanometer	Nitroglycerin	
Pulse oximeter	Labetalol	
Capnograph	Anesthetics	
IV cannulas	Fentanyl	
Syringes	Benzodiazepines	
	Pancuronium	
	Thiopental	
	Etomidate	

- Ensure the adequacy of arterial and venous cannulation.
- Check for hemostasis.
- Connect the portable monitoring devices to the electric outlet.
- Monitor cardiopulmonary values during the manipulation of organs (heart, lung, major vessels) at the moment of introduction and positioning of the IORT applicator cone to encompass the tumor bed.

3.2.6.4 Considerations During IORT

In thoracic surgery, an oxygen (50%) and nitrous oxide (50%) mixture is used for anesthetic maintenance during IORT. Supplementary doses of (fentanyl and pancuronium are given if necessary. In abdominal surgery, and depending on blood arterial pressure, an oxygen (70%) and enflurane (30%) mixture is used.

Immediately before the radiation exposure, all attendant personnel withdraw from the radiotherapy unit. A close circuit audiovisual system, including two television cameras in the treatment room, allows surveillance of the patient and the monitoring devices in the control area. One camera views the patient and the location of the treatment tube, while the other is zoomed toward the anesthesia machine and the monitoring devices (Fig. 3.2). The mean duration of exposure to radiation has been 6 min (range 2.5–20 min).

3.2.6.5 Consideration After IORT

Before the patient is redraped, the hemostasis of the tumor bed is check. The patient is then transported back to the operating room, where the surgical procedure is completed.

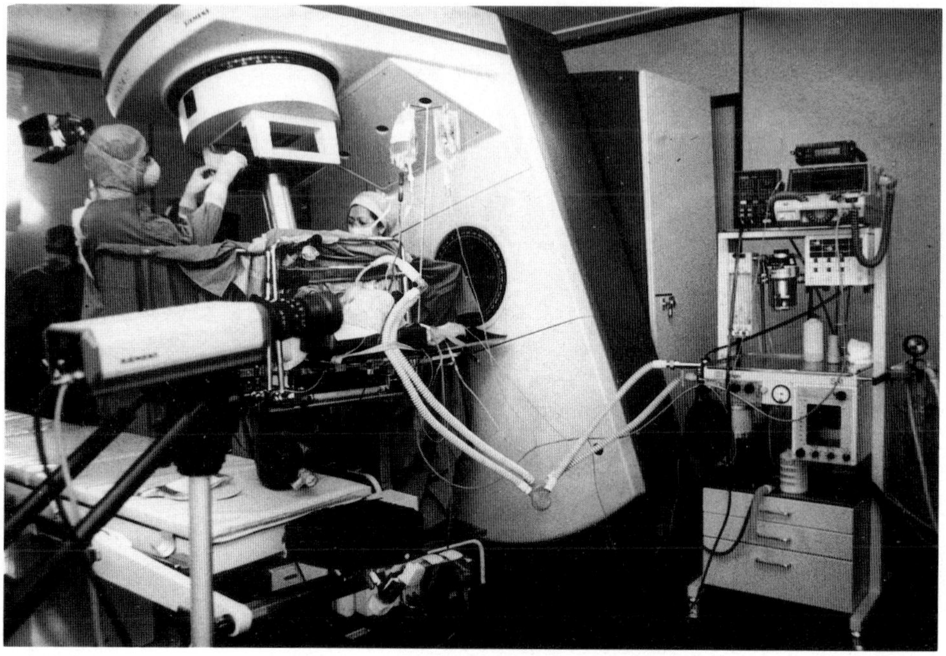

Fig. 3.2. Patient monitoring during preparation for IORT

3.2.7 Post-IORT Evaluation

In the operating room, after reconnection to the main monitoring instruments and ventilation systems, analytical blood determinations (hemoglobin, hematocrit, total proteins, electrolytes, arterial blood gases) for baseline are performed and replacement therapy is introduced if required. After surgery, the patient is transported to the ICU, where he or she is supported with controlled ventilation for approximately 6–12 h.

3.3 Complications

In 468 IORT procedures only two serious complications have been observed: an accidental endotracheal extubation, and an acute massive hemorrhage due to accidental release of a clamped blood vessel during manipulation of the IORT field. Both were readily managed and resolved.

There have been no complications directly attributable to anesthesia. In some instances it was necessary to interrupt the radiation treatment temporarily in order to deal with minor problems.

The most frequent complications have been diffuse hemorrhage of tumor beds after very aggressive surgery with insufficient hemostasis. No such cases have resulted in significant hemodynamic compromise.

Another interesting aspect is the low rate of infections during the postsurgical period, which is similar to the infection rates following less aggressive surgery in non-IORT patients.

In conclusion, IORT has proven to be a feasible treatment modality which can be used with minimum risk provided a careful operation is planned and close cooperation exists among surgeons, anesthesiologists, radiotherapists, physicists, and nurses (HOLLON 1989).

References

Bashein G, Russell AH, Momii ST (1986) Anesthesia and remote monitoring for intraoperative radiation therapy. Anesthesiology 64: 804–807

Friesen RH, Morrison JE Jr, Verbrugge JJ, Daniel WE, Aarestad NO, Burrington JD (1987) Anesthesia for intraoperative radiation therapy in children. J Surg Oncol 35: 96–98

Hodel PE, Martin JT (1989) Anesthesiologic considerations of intraoperative radiation therapy. In: Dobelbower RR, Abe M (eds) Intraoperative radiation therapy. CRC, Boca Raton, Fl, pp 75–82

Hollon AD (1989) Nursing and technological considerations in intraoperative radiation therapy. In: Dobelbower RR, Abe M (eds) Intraoperative radiation therapy. CRC, Boca Raton, Fl, pp 83–88

4 Intracranial Tumors

Felipe A. Calvo, Oscar Abuchaibe, Vicente Vanaclocha, and Francisco Aguilera

CONTENTS

4.1 Introduction 31
4.2 Previous Experiences 32
4.2.1 Tissue Tolerance Studies 32
4.2.2 Clinical Results 32
4.3 Treatment Protocol 33
4.3.1 Primary Disease 33
4.3.2 Recurrent Disease 33
4.4 Analysis of Results 33
4.4.1 Patient, Tumor, and Treatment Characteristics 34
4.4.2 Toxicity and Complications 34
4.4.3 Patterns of Disease Progression 35
4.4.4 Survival Data 35
4.5 Conclusion 35
References 35

4.1 Introduction

The role of radiation therapy in tumors of the central nervous system is well known, and in most tumor types it is an important modality in the overall therapeutic strategy. (Karlson and Brady 1987). In the case of primary tumors of the central nervous system the most frequent cause of treatment failure is local recurrence. Therefore, there is a need to improve the use of local treatment modalities such as surgery and radiation therapy, or the combination of both. The conventional treatment of high grade astrocytomas has combined surgery and brain irradiation, as well as including chemotherapy with nitrosureas (Levin et al. 1989). This histologic subtype is the most frequent brain tumor, and the final treatment results have reached a plateau since the last decade. Multi-institutional randomized trials exploring several treatment programs, including variations in chemotherapy regimes and radiotherapy schemes, have constantly reported median survival times of around 12 months, with a small proportion of patients displaying long-term survival (Shapiro 1986). An important feature of prospective trials has been the identification of favorable prognostic factors in patients with high grade astrocytoma, such as an age of less than 40 years, the histologic subtype anaplastic foci astrocytoma, and excellence of surgery (Nelson et al. 1982).

Radiotherapy trials have examined the relationship between local tumor control and total radiation dose (Walker et al. 1979). In most solid tumors it is reasonable to state that local tumor control is a dose-related feature. In primary neoplasms of the central nervous system the radiation dose is limited by the tolerance of normal brain tissue. Contemporary means of increasing total radiation doses in areas at risk for residual disease are the use of either altered fractionation schedules (exploiting repair processes in normal tissues) or sophisticated boosting techniques able to deliver high doses of radiation in small volumes. IORT is an attractive technique that warrants investigation as a boosting modality in brain tumor patients undergoing surgery. Tumors located in the periphery of the cerebral hemispheres can be removed and an electron beam can treat the surgical bed or any area of residual disease. IORT will prevent a significant part of the contralateral brain from receiving radiation, and at the same time very accurate evaluation of the areas of residual disease can be performed during the neurosurgical procedure. Although the integration of IORT in the management of brain tumor patients seems attractive and relatively simple, there are several technical limitations. The craniotomy incision has to be large to facilitate positioning of the IORT cone, and following tumor resection a cavity is left so that a decision on whether to use bolus material in the area has to be taken.

Felipe A. Calvo, Dr., Director and Consultant, Oscar Abuchaibe, Dr., Radiotherapy Division, Department of Oncology, Clinica Universitaria de Navarra, 31080 Pamplona, Spain

Vicente Vanaclocha, Dr., Consultant, Francisco Aguilera, Dr., Director, Neurosurgery Division, Clinica Universitaria de Navarra, 31080 Pamplona Spain

The general indications for IORT also pertain to tumor histologies other than high grade astrocytomas, such as meningiomas and low grade astrocytomas with a supratentorial or peripheral location.

The final treatment program (radiation dose, volume, etc.) has to be individualized. Central lesions and tumors of the posterior fossa are difficult to treat by IORT due to technical limitations. i.e., inadequate tumor exposure or difficult transport of the patient.

4.2 Previous Experiences

4.2.1 Tissue Tolerance Studies

There is a lack of information regarding the tolerance of normal brain tissue to high single doses of electron beams, such as are used in IORT, both with and without supplementary fractionated external beam radiotherapy. This is an area of interest for research. It is known that peripheral nerves are extremely sensitive to IORT, which has been an unexpected finding in the clinical and basic research on this treatment modality (Kinsella et al. 1984; Le Coteur et al. 1989). It seems that damage to peripheral nerves induced by IORT is a dose-related feature and a threshold dose has been suggested (Kinsella et al. 1988). Nevertheless, the data obtained in animal experiments and clinical research regarding peripheral nerve tolerance to IORT cannot be extrapolated to the human brain. A further problem is the selection of the best animal model to use when testing brain tolerance to IORT; a monkey model might be preferable to a dog model.

4.2.2 Clinical Results

Several clinical studies have reported results in brain tumor patients treated with IORT. Neurosurgical considerations regarding the integration of this modality in the management of tumors of the central nervous system suggest the following to be important components of an "optimal protocol": (a) maximal surgical removal of the tumor; (b) an adequate interval between initial surgery and reopening for IORT; (c) a reasonably superficial tumor location, and (d) inclusion of the areas of residual disease within the electron beam, plus a margin of normal tissue (Greenblatt and Rayport 1989). The same authors, however, reported only one case in which such an optimal protocol could be employed. Variations on the use of IORT in brain tumor patients have included: IORT at the time of initial surgery (Goldson et al. 1984); IORT for recurrent malignant gliomas (Abe et al. 1980; Yamashita et al. 1985); repeat application of IORT (Terao 1982; Greenblatt and Rayport 1989); and IORT for metastatic disease (Greenblatt and Rayport 1989; Matsutani 1989), including an exceptional case of metastatic melanoma to the posterior fossa.

The available medical literature on the use of IORT in intracranial tumors relates only to small series of patients and anecdotal cases from which it is scarcely possible to draw definitive conclusions on efficacy and toxicity. The largest published clinical experience is from Japan (Matsutani 1989). This author has described the results in three consecutive pilot studies comprising 32 adult patients with malignant glioma (24 not previously treated and 8 recurrent) and 20 with brain metastases (18 solitary and 2 multiple). In general the treatment protocol involved the use of IORT as a boosting modality in combination with external beam irradiation. In the first of the pilot studies, brain edema developed in two of three cases treated with IORT doses in the range of 25–30 Gy, without external beam radiotherapy. The second pilot study did not show brain edema in patients treated with 15–20 Gy and external beam radiotherapy. The final study, involving 15 patients and better selection of cases, reported seven patients still to be alive, with follow-up ranging from 6 months to 9 years. The longest survivor in this group had been treated three different times with IORT. In cases of recurrent glioblastoma the median time to tumor progression was 30 weeks. Among the 20 patients with brain metastases, ten were alive at the time of the report (follow-up ranging from 5+ to 34+ months). It is interesting to note that the IORT cone diameter ranged from 2 to 6 cm, but a large proportion of procedures were performed with 3- and 4-cm cones. The only fatal treatment–related complication reported was a case of postoperative brain edema.

Further clinical information from Japanese investigators is available with respect to 27 cases of high grade astrocytoma treated with 15–50 Gy IORT plus external beam radiotherapy (30–52 Gy, mean dose 50 Gy) and ACNU chemotherapy (Yanagawa et al. 1989). Survival rates at 1 and 2 years were 88% and 40%, respectively. The data compared favorably with the results in a similar group of patients not treated with IORT. No adverse effects were noted. MATSUTANI updated his series by analyzing 22 patients with nonrecurrent glioblastoma treated with external beam irradiation (35–80 Gy, median 70 Gy) and a 10–20 Gy IORT boost. The median time to tumor progression was 60 weeks, with 1- and 2-year survival rates of 100% and 61%, respectively. Seven patients were alive and disease free with follow-up ranging from 26 to 192 weeks (MATSUTANI and TANAKA 1989). Finally, at Kyoto University there were three long-term survivors (follow-up from 36 to 74 months) among 13 patients with recurrent malignant brain tumors who underwent further surgery and IORT (YAMASHITA et al. 1989).

In the United States a pilot study was performed and reported by the group at Howard University (GOLDSON et al. 1984). The treatment protocol consisted in surgery, 15 Gy IORT, and 50 Gy external beam irradiation in 25 fractions, with an additional 5 Gy cone down boost to the tumor bed. There were a miscellaneous group of histologies including glioblastoma multiforme, anaplastic astrocytomas, oligodendrogliomas, meningiomas, and mixed histologies. Tumor location was predominantly hemispheric, the exceptions being two cases involving the posterior fossa and one, the thalamus. At the time of publication six patients were alive and disease free; four had had malignant astrocytomas (follow-up of 10–15 months) and two, meningiomas (follow-up of 33 and 42 months). Among the IORT-related complications described were two episodes of symptomatic cerebral edema, coma, and transient seizures, and one episode of bleeding requiring reexploration.

The clinical experiences reported using IORT in intracranial tumors seem to confirm that use of the modality is feasible in this disease site. Moderate to high doses of IORT appear to be acceptably tolerated, although acute brain edema has been described. A rigorous analysis of the possible benefit of the integration of this technique in the management of brain tumor patients is difficult on the basis of the available data, but there is agreement among experts that the initial clinical results are interesting.

4.3 Treatment Protocol

4.3.1 Primary Disease

The treatment protocol for patients not previously treated consisted in craniotomy, histologic confirmation of malignancy, and maximal surgical debulking. The areas of residual disease were identified by the neurosurgeon and radiotherapist together, and a decision was taken regarding the cone size to be used and the need (or lack of it) for bolus material in an effort to homogenize the radiation distribution in the postsurgical cavity.

The electron energy was selected according to the general rules employed in our program: the 90% isodose curve had to encompass completely the residual tumor or target volume with a 0.5- to 1-cm margin of theoretically normal brain. All patients not previously treated received 15 Gy to the target volume. External beam radiotherapy was added 4 weeks after surgery, using high energy photon beams (6–15 MV) and a parallel opposed field technique covering the whole brain, delivering a total dose of 50 Gy in 25 fractions. Three patients in this group received weekly intra-arterial cisplatin at the time of external irradiation (CALVO et al. 1989). No further chemotherapy or radiation therapy was given to these patients.

4.3.2 Recurrent Disease

Patients with evidence of tumor recurrence following radical external beam radiotherapy, good general and neurologic status, and peripheral hemispheric tumors were considered for reoperation and IORT boost. The total single dose ranged from 10 to 20 Gy depending upon the type of previous radiotherapy: those patients who had received high doses of external beam irradiation (65–70 Gy) received the lower doses of IORT (10 Gy). Technical details of IORT in these patients are similar to those described in respect of patients with primary disease. In this subgroup (i.e., patients with recurrent tumors), external beam radiotherapy after reoperation and IORT was omitted.

4.4 Analysis of Results

In a period of 5 years only ten patients with an established diagnosis of brain tumor have been treated with IORT. This is due in part to the existing competitive treatment programs for these patients in our institution. The analysis of the results observed in this small group of patients is reported in a summarized manner.

4.4.1 Patient, Tumor, and Treatment Characteristics

Of the ten patients, seven were males and three, females. Their ages ranged from 7 to 61 years with a mean of 37 years. Karnofsky performance status ranged from 40% to 100% (mean 60%). Tumor histology was reported as glioblastoma multiforme in two cases, astrocytoma grade III in four cases, and ependymoma, neuroblastoma, oligodendroglioma, and meningioma in one case each. Six patients had primary disease (not previously treated) and four, recurrent disease (previous radiotherapy). Following surgery, macroscopic residual tumor was present in all ten cases. The IORT cone diameter was 5 cm in all procedures, using a single field. The electron beam energy selected was 12 or 15 MeV in five cases, and 18 or 20 MeV in the remaining five cases. One patient received 10 Gy IORT, six were treated with 15 Gy, and three received 20 Gy. The external beam radiotherapy course was completed by the patients with primary disease, with total doses in the range of 45–60 Gy (Table 4.1).

Table 4.1. Characteristics of the series of intracranial tumor patients (n = 10) treated with IORT

	No. of patients
Sex	
Male	7
Female	3
Age	
Mean: 37 years	
Range: 7–61 years	
Karnofsky performance status	
Mean: 60%	
Range: 40%–100%	
Tumor Histology	
Glioblastoma multiforme	2
Astrocytoma grade III	4
Ependymoma	1
Neuroblastoma	1
Oligodendroglioma	1
Meningioma	1
Disease status	
Primary	6
Recurrent	4
Postsurgical residue	
Macroscopic	10
Microscopic	–
IORT cone diameter	
5 cm	10
IORT electron energy (MeV)	
12–15	5
18–20	5
IORT total dose (Gy)	
10	1
15	6
20	3
External beam radiotherapy (Gy)	
45	1
50–60	4

4.4.2 Toxicity and Complications

In this small group of patients only one complication related to IORT was observed. This was the development of brain edema in the postoperative period in a patient with the diagnosis of recurrent glioblastoma multiforme following external beam radiotherapy (the time interval free of tumor progression was 9 months), in whom a reoperation

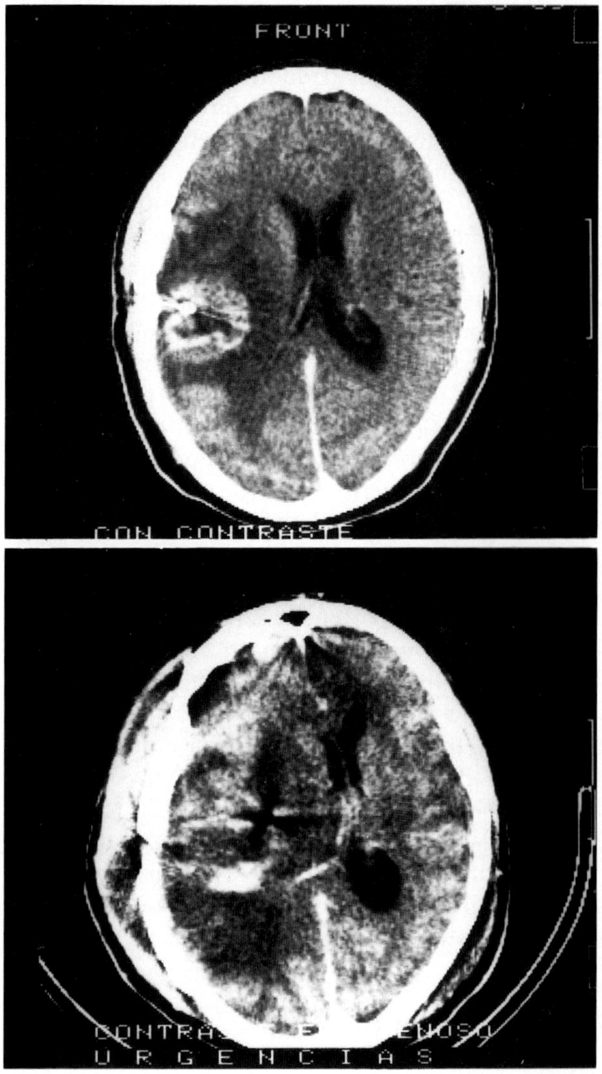

a

b

Fig. 4.1. Brain edema in a patient with recurrent glioblastoma multiforme: **a** preoperative CT scan; **b** CT scan 48 h following 20 Gy IORT

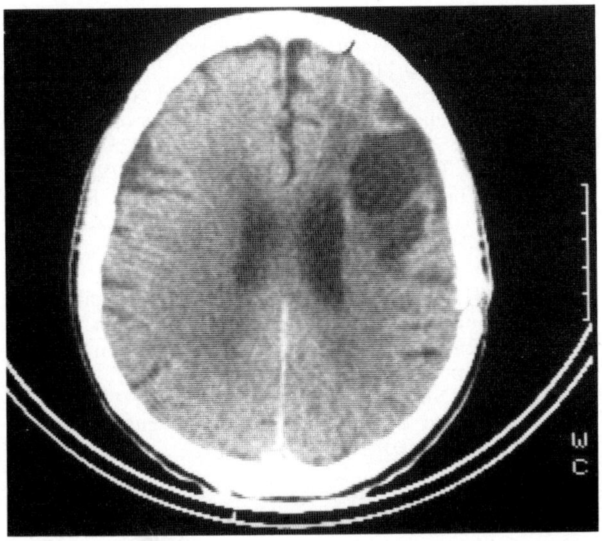

Fig. 4.2. Long-term changes in a patient with more than 4 years' survival. The area of hypodensity is clinically silent

was performed for surgical tumor debulking, plus 20 Gy IORT. During the first 48 h the patient deteriorated neurologically and a CT scan revealed significant brain edema in the homolateral hemisphere (Fig. 4.1). The patient was medically managed with steroids and antiedema measures, and recovered properly neurologically. This patient survived 10 months after his second operation and died suddenly (with the tumor stabilized) from an unknown cause. No autopsy was performed. No wound infections or postoperative fever were seen in this group. The longest survivor (more than 4 years' follow-up from IORT) has an excellent general status and is free of neurologic symptoms, with a CT scan showing a clinically silent area of hypodensity in the treated area (Fig. 4.2).

4.4.3 Patterns of Disease Progression

Nine patients could be analyzed for disease progression (one patient was lost to follow-up while free of recurrence at 6 months after IORT). Seven patients developed local failure, two of them with contralateral tumor involvement.

4.4.4 Survival Data

All patients with tumor progression have died. Two patients are still alive and free of disease at 10 and 56 months' follow-up. One had astrocytoma grade III and one a recurrent meningioma.

4.5 Conclusion

This review of our experience using IORT in the management of intracranial tumors does not allow definite conclusions to be drawn, except that the modality is feasible in this tumor site and that long-term survival can be observed. This confirms the findings of previous studies. The intracranial site is a further example of a disease site in which IORT's benefits can be exploited from the viewpoint of accuracy in the radiation boost and use of high dose radiotherapy at the time of surgical debulking. However, an important practical limitation of IORT in this tumor location is the small treatment zone that can be boosted (usually less than 5 cm in diameter). Due to the inconveniences of the technique and the paucity of available clinical data, it will be a long time before IORT can be considered a valuable technique deserving of exploration in phase III trials by cooperative groups or multi-institutional trials.

References

Abe M, Takahashi M, Yabumoto E, Adchi H, Voshii M, Mori K (1980) Clinical experiences with intraoperative radiotherapy for locally advanced cancers. Cancer 45: 40–48

Calvo FA, Dy C, Henriquez I et al. (1989) Simultaneous cisplatinum and radiotherapy for the treatment of malignant glioma. Radiother Oncol 14: 83–88

Goldson AL, Streeter OE, Ashayeri E, Collier-Manning J, Barber JB, Fan KJ (1984) Intraoperative radiotherapy for intracranial malignancies. Cancer 54: 2807–2813

Greenblatt SH, Rayport M (1989) Neurosurgical considerations in intraoperative radiation therapy. In: Dobelbower RR, Abe M (eds) Intraoperative radiation therapy. CRC, Boca Raton, Fl, pp 123–136

Karlson U, Brady LW (1987) Primary intracranial neoplasms. In: Perez CA, Brady LW (eds) Principles and practice of radiation oncology. JB Lippincott, Philadelphia, pp 408–436

Kinsella TJ, Sindelar WF, de Luca AM, Terrill R (1984) Tolerance of peripheral nerve to intraoperative radiotherapy (IORT): clinical and experimental studies. Int J Radiat Oncol Biol Phys 10 [Suppl 2]: 80

Kinsella TJ, Sindelar WF, de Luca AM (1988) Threshold dose for peripheral nerve injury following intraoperative radiotherapy (IORT) in a large animal model. Int J Radiat Oncol Biol Phys 15 [Suppl 1]: 205

Le Coteur RA, Gillette EL, Powers BE et al. (1989) Peripheral neuropathies following experimental intraoperative radiation therapy (IORT). Int J Radiat Oncol Biol Phys 17: 583–590

Levin VA, Sheline GE, Gutin PH (1989) Neoplasms of the central nervous system. In: De Vita VT, Hellman S, Rosemberg SA (eds) Principles and practice of oncology. JB Lippincott, Philadelphia, pp 1557–1611
Matsutani M (1989) Intraoperative radiation therapy for malignant brain tumors. In: Dobelbower RR, Abe M (eds) Intraoperative radiation therapy. CRC, Boca Raton, Fl, pp 137–158
Matsutani M, Tanaka Y (1989) Intraoperative radiation therapy (IORT) for cerebral glioblastoma. Strahlenther Onkol 165: 781
Matsutani M, Matsuda T, Nagashima T (1984) Surgical treatment and radiation therapy for glioblastoma multiforme with special reference to intraoperative radiotherapy: Jpn J Cancer Res 30: 201–209
Nelson DF, Nelson JS, Davis DR (1982) Survival and prognosis of patients with astrocytoma with atypical or anaplastic features. J Neurooncol 11: 776–780
Shapiro WR (1986) Therapy of adult malignant brain tumors: What have the clinical trials taught us?. Semin Oncol 13: 38–45
Terao H (1982) Intraoperative radiotherapy and conformation radiotherapy for malignant brain tumors. Neo Skinkei Geka 10:119–127
Walker MD, Strike TA, Sheline GE (1979) An analysis of dose-effect relationship in the radiotherapy of malignant gliomas. Int J Radiat Oncol Biol Phys 5: 1725–1731
Yamashita J, Handa H, Keyaki A, Abe M (1985) Indication for intraoperative radiation therapy (IOR) in the treatment of recurrent malignant gliomas. American Association of Neurological Surgeons. Atlanta (April 21–25)
Yamashita J, Kikuchi H, Abe M, Takahashi M, Shibamoto Y (1989) Indication of intraoperative radiation therapy for the treatment of recurrent malignant brain tumors. Strahlenther Onkol 165: 781
Yanagawa S, Doi H, Sakai N, Yamada H (1989) Intraoperative radiation therapy (IORT) of malignant gliomas. Strahlenther Onkol 165: 781

5 Head and Neck Cancer

FELIPE A. CALVO, OSCAR ABUCHAIBE, JOSÉ MARÍA SERRA, and RAFAEL GARCÍA-TAPIA

CONTENTS

5.1	Introduction	37
5.2	Previous Experiences	38
5.2.1	Tissue Tolerance Studies	38
5.2.2	Clinical Results	38
5.3	Treatment Protocol	39
5.4	Results	39
5.4.1	Patient, Tumor, and Treatment Characteristics	39
5.4.2	Patterns of Recurrence	40
5.4.3	Outcome and Survival	40
5.5	Conclusion	40
	References	41

5.1 Introduction

The possible role of IORT in the management of head and neck tumors has rarely been explored, an exception being the large series at the Methodist Hospital of Indiana (GARRETT et al. 1989). IORT can be introduced in the multidisciplinary management of head and neck cancer as a boosting modality in areas of residual disease or close surgical margins in patients with locally advanced tumor, in an effort to promote local tumor control. The potential advantages of IORT in these tumor locations do not derive from normal tissue sparing, but from better definition of high risk areas for recurrence and the simultaneous combination of high dose radiotherapy and surgical debulking.

The conventional management of head and neck cancer patients varies according to tumor stage and site of origin. In early tumor stages radical radiotherapy is regarded as a treatment option able to preserve the anatomy and adequate function of the different organs. In intermediate tumor stages the combination of surgery and radiation therapy is in most cases considered the best alternative to assure disease control. Finally, patients with locally advanced disease patients might be considered candidates for investigational treatment protocols due to their poor prognosis. Locoregional recurrences are the most common cause of failure, particularly in advanced nodal disease of the neck. The results of surgery and external beam radiotherapy in the treatment of head and neck cancer patients have generally reached a plateau, although certain technical advances in both modalities have allowed improved treatment in selected patients. These advances comprise the introduction of reconstructive surgical procedures and myocutaneous flaps, and the availability of electron beam and brachytherapy techniques for sophisticated radiation boost in the areas of large tumor burden (MILLION et al. 1989).

Recurrent disease following radical treatment is an important problem in head and neck cancer patients. In most cases it is a desperate situation in which no treatment alternative can be found. Nevertheless, occasionally patients can be selected for rescue therapy, and some cases of long-term survival are known. In selecting such patients it is necessary to evaluate carefully the clinical features and previous treatments, as well as the skills and the results obtained in each institution.

An interesting suggestion concerning the use of IORT in head and neck cancer patients was that myocutaneous flaps be used in patients undergoing radical dissection for locally advanced or recurrent neck disease. In these cases the area primarily at risk for residual tumor is the major vessels (carotid artery and internal jugular vein), but the skin might also be contaminated by neoplastic tissue. A myocutaneous flap might add some security margin to the surgical resection, avoid recontamination of the IORT-treated area, and allow some additional external beam irradiation even in patients previously treated.

FELIPE A. CALVO, Dr., Director and Consultant, OSCAR ABUCHAIBE, Dr., Radiotherapy Division, Department of Oncology, JOSÉ M. SERRA, Consultant, Department of Reconstructive and Plastic Surgery, RAFAEL GARCIA-TAPIA, Dr., Consultant, Department of Otorhinolaryngology, Clinica Universitaria de Navarra, 31080 Pamplona, Spain

5.2 Previous Experiences

5.2.1 Tissue Tolerance Studies

The normal tissues included in IORT for head and neck cancer patients are in general those left in situ after radical neck dissection: major vessels, subcutaneous tissues, peripheral nerves, muscle, vertebral bodies, and rarely the esophagus and pharyngeal wall mucosa and its sutures. Several studies in animal models have investigated the tolerance of these tissues to IORT alone or in combination with external beam radiotherapy. In general the results can be summarized by saying that the peripheral nerve is the dose-limiting structure both for IORT alone and for IORT in combination with external beam radiotherapy, and that the remaining structures tolerate reasonable doses in the range of 10–15 Gy plus full course conventional external beam irradiation (50 Gy) or a 20 Gy single IORT dose (Le Coteur et al. 1989; Powers et al. 1989a,b; Gillette et al. 1988).

One experimental study employing a canine model analyzed tissue changes after IORT in the cervical area (Mittal et al. 1989). The experiment was designed to deliver escalating doses of IORT (25, 35, 45, and 55 Gy) through an 8-cm cone to a treatment zone including a portion of the carotid artery, the internal jugular vein, and the vagus nerve. Animals were sacrificed 3 and 6 months after IORT. Carotid rupture was not observed in any of the animals. In both vessels an increased collagen content was seen in the tunica media. The vagus nerve showed severe demyelination and loss of fibers, these changes appearing to be dose dependent.

5.2.2 Clinical Results

The experience at the Methodist Hospital of Indiana is the most relevant clinical experience using IORT in head and neck cancer patients and has been updated several times (Garrett et al. 1987, 1989). In their last report (Freeman et al. 1990) a total of 104 patients treated in a period of 6 years were available for analysis. Tumor histologies included in the study were: squamous cell carcinoma (74), salivary gland carcinoma (24), sarcomas (3), melanoma (2), and recurrent basal cell carcinoma (1). Forty patients were treated with surgery and IORT as the initial treatment, and 64 in a bid to rescue previous treatment. IORT dose ranged from 15 to 20 Gy with the exception of one case treated with 100 Gy to the mandible. The cone sizes most frequently used were 4.5 and 6 cm in diameter. The neck was the predominant treatment zone in 38 patients. The analysis of patterns of tumor progression for squamous cell carcinoma showed an overall local control rate of 40% with minor differences between groups subclassified by postsurgical residual disease: microscopic residual disease had a local control rate of 44%, close surgical margins 30%, and gross residual disease 43%. Twenty-five autopsies were performed in patients who died with local disease. In 22 patients, the local recurrence was found to be marginal to the treatment field. Local tumor control in the group of salivary gland neoplasms was obtained in 88% of cases. Several complications were related to IORT, including six cases of osteoradionecrosis (all patients were treated with external beam radiotherapy, and in three cases the mandible was not included in the IORT field), six large fistulas reconstructed with flaps (three in previously irradiated patients), and three cases of carotid or innominate artery rupture (one at the time of tumor recurrence).

Adopting a systematic approach in both recurrent and primary disease, this large series has established the feasibility of IORT during head and neck cancer surgery. The pattern of disease progression does not appear to correlate with local tumor control rates and postsurgical residual disease, but this has to be analyzed further due to the heterogeneity of disease status (primary versus recurrent, differing tumor stage, etc.) and treatment protocol. An important aspect to emerge from the study is the need to consider as a protocol requirement the use of large treatment cones in all cases, trying to include not only the area of evident residual disease but also a margin of normal tissue. The identification of treatment complications, mainly grouped in recurrent patients, constitutes valuable information.

Schmitt et al. (1989) have reported preliminary results regarding the use of IORT in cases of T3–T4 squamous cell carcinoma of the base of the tongue. In all 15 patients treated (five recurrent cases) surgery was able to remove gross tumor completely. The IORT boost dose was 20 Gy in 13 cases and 17.5 Gy in two cases. Treatment cones were 4 and 5 cm in diameter. Ten patients received a full course of fractionated external

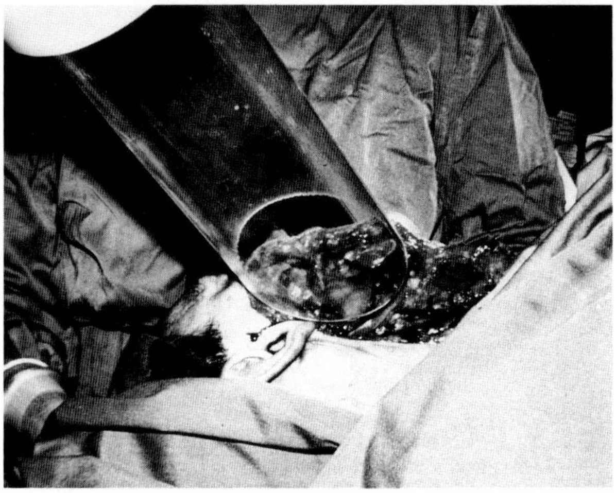

Fig. 5.1. Example of an IORT procedure in a patient with recurrent head and neck cancer

beam radiotherapy (50–56 Gy). The follow-up of these patients at the time of publication ranged from 6 to more than 12 months. Both T4 cases with microscopic residual disease after surgery had a local recurrence confirmed in the 3rd month of follow-up. Two additional recurrences were noted in the floor of the mouth at 8 and 10 months after surgery. No postoperative or delayed complications were observed.

5.3 Treatment Protocol

In the Clinica Universitaria de Navarra IORT was part of the initial treatment approach in only 4 of 17 patients with squamous cell carcinoma of the head and neck. For this reason, the treatment program was designed on an individualized basis, adopting a combined treatment strategy for rescue of recurrent disease in each patient.

In all cases attempts were made to perform maximal surgical debulking. The use of myocutaneous flaps soon became an important component of the surgical protocol. The indication for use of myocutaneous flaps was either tumor involvement of the skin or previous radiotherapy compromising tissue healing and rendering inappropriate further external beam irradiation.

Intraoperative radiation therapy was given to the areas of known residual disease or areas at high risk for recurrence, generally using large treatment cones. The beam energy was selected to treat adequately the tissue thickness with a margin which had to be included in the 90% isodose curve. The dose ranged from 5 to 20 Gy (Fig. 5.1).

Fractionated external beam radiotherapy was delivered in those cases in which it appeared to be safe, taking into consideration tissue changes due to previous irradiation and the presence of new tissue in the area (myocutaneous flap). Mixed beams of photons and electrons were used in accordance with tumor origin and site of recurrence. Fractionation was the conventional 2 Gy 5 times per week, and in all cases total doses reached 45–50 Gy.

5.4 Results

5.4.1 Patient, Tumor, and Treatment Characteristics

In the period analyzed (1984–1989), 17 patients with an established diagnosis of squamous cell carcinoma of the head and neck were treated with IORT. Their ages ranged from 35 to 78 years (median 58 years). Fourteen were males and three, females. Karnofsky performance status was 70% or more in 12 patients. Disease was recurrent in 13 patients, nine of whom had undergone previous surgery and radiotherapy (Table 5.1). Surgery was able to remove all macroscopic tumor in six cases, but left macroscopic residual disease in 11. Myocutaneous flaps were used in 12 cases (all recurrent following previous radiotherapy). Fractionated external beam irradiation was given preoperatively in two patients and postoperatively in 11; it was omitted in four. The IORT single

Table 5.1. Patient and tumor characteristics in IORT for head and neck cancer (n = 17)

	No. of patients
Age	
Range: 35–78 years	
Median: 58 years	
Sex	
Male	14
Female	3
Karnofsky performance status	
≤70%	12
>70%	5
Disease status	
Primary	4
Recurrent	13
Previous radiotherapy	9
Locally advanced	7

Table 5.2. Treatment characteristics regarding disease status (primary vs recurrent)

	Primary disease	Recurrent disease
Surgery		
Macroscopic residual disease	1	5
Microscopic residual disease	3	8
Myocutaneous flap	4	8
Radiotherapy		
Preoperative	1	1
Postoperative	2	9
Not given	1	3
IORT		
Cone diameter (cm)		
5–6	1	7
7–8	1	1
9–12	3	8
Electron energy (MeV)		
6–9	4	8
12–20	1	5
Total dose (Gy)		
5	–	2
10	2	3
15	2	7
20	–	1
Number of fields		
Single	3	10
Multiple	1	3

dose was 10–15 Gy in 14 cases, while two patients received 5 Gy in situations in which multiple fields were appropriate and some overlapping between fields was suspected. One patient received 20 Gy over an area of known macroscopic residual disease (Table 5.2).

5.4.2 Patterns of Recurrence

The first site of disease progression has been carefully analyzed. Local recurrence alone, in the head and neck area, has been seen in seven patients (all recurrent cases). Combined local and distant progression was observed in three cases, and in no case was a distant site the first and only site of failure. At the time of this analysis seven patients were free of any recurrence. All local failures were located in the neck, and five were seen in patients with macroscopic residual disease after surgery (Table 5.3).

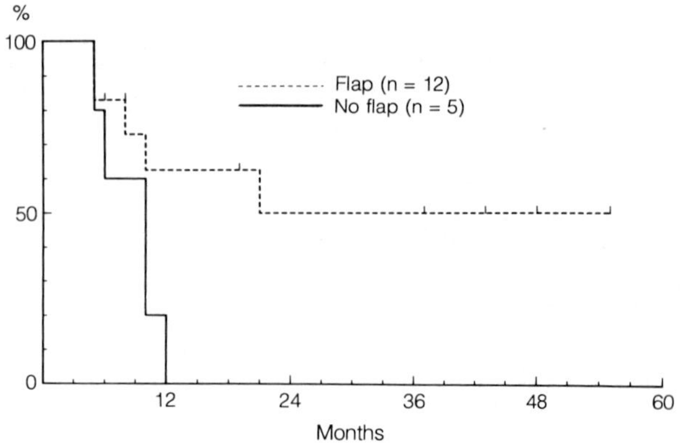

Fig. 5.2. Actuarial survival curves for patients treated with IORT for head and neck cancer

Table 5.3. Patterns of tumor progression

Disease status	Local failure	Local failure + distant metastasis	Distant metastasis
Primary	–	1	–
Recurrent	7	2	–
Total	7	3	–

5.4.3 Outcome and Survival

As mentioned above, seven patients are alive and free of disease while ten have died due to tumor recurrence. There are no surviving patients in the group in which myocutaneous flaps were not used (Table 5.4). Actuarial survival curves are shown in Fig. 5.2.

5.5 Conclusion

Intraoperative radiation therapy in head and neck cancer is an attractive radiotherapy boosting modality worthy of further exploration. Analysis of

Table 5.4. Local control and outcome according to type of surgery

Type of surgery	No. of patients	Median follow-up (months)	Local control	Patient status Alive/dead
Myocutaneous flap	12	14.5+	7	7/5
No flap	5	10	–	–/5
Total	17	12	7	7/10

the published data and our own experience does not completely clarify the role of this technique. Local tumor control has been achieved even in patients with residual tumor after surgery and/ or recurrent disease. Although head and neck cancers are common in oncologic practice, IORT trials have to compete with many other studies of combined modality therapy including chemotherapy and other forms of radiation therapy.

References

Freeman SB, Hamaker RC, Singer MI, Pugh N, Garrett P, Ross D (1990) Intraoperative radiotherapy of head and neck cancer. Arch Otolaryngol Head Neck Surg 116: 165–168

Garrett P, Pugh N, Ross D et al. (1987) Intraoperative radiation therapy for advanced or recurrent head and neck cancer. Int J Radiat Oncol Biol Phys 13: 785–788

Garrett P, Pugh N, Ross D, Hamaker R, Singer M (1989) Intraoperative radiation therapy for advanced or recurrent head and neck malignancies. In: Dobelbower RR, Abe M (eds) Intraoperative radiation therapy. CRC, Boca Raton, Fl, pp 155–164

Gillette EL, Powers BE, McChesney SL et al. (1988) Response of aorta and branch arteries to experimental intraoperative irradiation. Int J Radiat Oncol Biol Phys 15 [Suppl 1]: 202

Hamaker RC, Singer MI, Pugh N et al. (1985) Management of the N3 neck: intraoperative radiation. Head Neck Cancer 1: 162–166

Le Coteur RA, Gillette EL, Powers BE et al. (1989) Peripheral neuropathies following experimental intraoperative irradiation. Int J Radiat Oncol Biol Phys 17: 583–590

Million RR, Cassisi NJ, Clark JR (1989) Cancer of the head and neck. In: De Vita VT, Hellman S, Rosemberg SA (eds) Cancer. Principles and practice of oncology, 3rd edn. JB Lippincott, Philadelphia, pp 488–590

Mittal BB, Pelzer H, Tsao CC et al. (1989) IORT of canine carotid artery, internal jugular vein and vagus nerve: application in the management of advanced head and neck cancer. Strahlenther Onkol 165: 768

Powers BE, Gillette EL, McChesney SL et al. (1989a) Muscle injury following experimental intraoperative irradiation. Int J Radiat Oncol Biol Phys 17 [Suppl 1]: 246

Powers BE, Gillette EL, McChesney SL et al. (1989b) Bone necrosis and tumor induction following experimental intraoperative irradiation. Int J Radiat Oncol Biol Phys 17: 559–567

Schmitt T, Puel G, Prades JM, Barbet M, Perron X, Mere P (1989) Intraoperative radiotherapy (IORT) for locally advanced carcinoma of the base of the tongue. Ann Radiol 32: 505–508

6 Lung Cancer

Felipe A. Calvo, David Ortiz de Urbina, Jesús Herreros, and Rafael Llorens

CONTENTS

6.1	Introduction	43
6.2	Previous Experiences	44
6.2.1	Tissue Tolerance Studies	44
6.2.2	Clinical Results	45
6.3	Treatment Protocol	45
6.3.1	Surgery	45
6.3.2	IORT	46
6.3.3	External Beam Radiotherapy	46
6.3.4	Chemotherapy	46
6.4	Analysis of Results	46
6.4.1	General Aspects of the Series	46
6.4.2	Toxicity and Complications	47
6.4.3	Patterns of Relapse	49
6.4.4	Survival Data	49
6.5	Conclusion	50
	References	50

6.1 Introduction

Locally advanced lung cancer represents a common disease in daily medical activity, and its poor prognosis is well known. Investigational therapeutic programs are needed to increase both median survival time and overall survival rates (Richards and Scarantino 1985). Stage III non-small cell lung cancer is considered a disease stage that will have a marginal benefit from surgery. In most cases residual disease will be left in the mediastinum and/or chest wall, or tumor resection cannot be performed at all. External beam radiotherapy may induce tumor regression and stabilization for some months in unresectable lesions, but local control rates in the long term are modest. Combined treatment with surgery and radiotherapy is the conventional recommendation in positive mediastinal node patients, and even in negative cases, in an effort to control thoracic disease progression. At the present time none of the above-mentioned treatment approaches have shown definitive evidence of improved survival in randomized studies, but there is a suggestion that thoracic tumor control is a dose-related feature (Emami and Perez 1987). Adjuvant chemotherapy has been extensively investigated, and its role in the management of this disease might be of interest in certain situations (Holmes and Gail 1986). Neoadjuvant chemotherapy is an attractive approach that might improve tumor resectability and survival rates (Martini et al. 1987).

The pattern of disease progression in lung cancer shows a high rate of combined local and systemic failures. In 30%–40% of patients the cause of death is related to thoracic complications due to uncontrolled locoregional disease (Cox 1983). Despite this dismal picture there is still a place for the development of intensified locoregional and systemic investigational treatment programs to improve results. Thoracic tumor control rates might benefit from the combination of surgery and radiotherapy. Surgical resection rates may be increased by neoadjuvant chemotherapy and preoperative external beam radiotherapy. Sophisticated boosting techniques, such as brachytherapy and IORT, would achieve higher doses in the areas of residual disease and therefore promote local tumor control. Systemic tumor progression might be prevented by more active chemotherapy regimes, at the moment available only for patients with chemosensitive tumors.

Small cell lung cancer is a well-recognized entity with a better prognosis that varies according to the tumor stage at the time of diagnosis. Some long-term survivors are seen, and the use of intensive alternating chemotherapy regimes is mandatory. Thoracic and prophylactic brain irradiation has to be considered in responding patients with localized disease (Litcher et al. 1985).

Felipe A. Calvo, Dr., Director and Consultant, David Ortiz de Urbina, Dr., Radiotherapy Division, Department of Oncology, Clinica Universitaria de Navarra, 31080 Pamplona, Spain

Jesús Herreros, Dr., Consultant, Rafael Llorens, Dr., Consultant, Department of Cardiovascular and Thoracic Surgery, 31080 Pamplona, Spain

Indications for and initial results of IORT during lung cancer surgery in our institution have been reported previously (Calvo et al. 1990). IORT can deliver a boost dose to areas of residual tumor in the mediastinum, chest wall, and hilum and to unresectable central tumors (Fig. 6.1). A combination of treatment zones can be decided upon at the time of the surgical procedure. The initial analysis of our experience showed clearly that IORT is feasible during lung cancer surgery and that large thoracic volumes can be adequately treated. From the beginning the protocol called for the use of moderate IORT total doses (10 Gy and occasionally 15 Gy), and the clinical tolerance of the whole treatment program has been acceptable. The surgeons have consistently adopted a positive attitude to IORT, resulting in a rapid accrual of patients to the protocol. The surgical incision is done on an individualized basis to facilitate IORT. The development of pleural or vascularized flaps to protect the bronchial stump when this is included in the IORT field is a new surgical maneuver first described in our institution. The following discussion is an update of the IORT experience obtained in lung cancer patients over a 5-year period.

6.2 Previous Experiences

6.2.1 Tissue Tolerance Studies

Information on the tolerance of mediastinal and thoracic viscera to IORT has been acquired from experimental animal studies using large dog models, with and without surgical tissue manipulation. In a dose escalation study using 20, 30, and 40 Gy in an IORT field which included collapsed lung parenchyma, esophagus, trachea, phrenic nerve, right atrium, and blood vessels, pathologic changes were observed at 30 Gy in the trachea and esophagus, with severe ulceration and peribronchial and perivascular chronic inflammation in the normal lung. A dose of 20 Gy produced minimal changes in the esophagus, trachea, and phrenic nerve, but major vessels and the atrium showed medial and adventitial fibrosis, obliterative endarteritis of the vasa vasorum, and severe coagulative necrosis. Acute pneumonitis was seen at all doses, and changes in the contralateral lung were detected using 12 MeV electrons (Barnes et al. 1987).

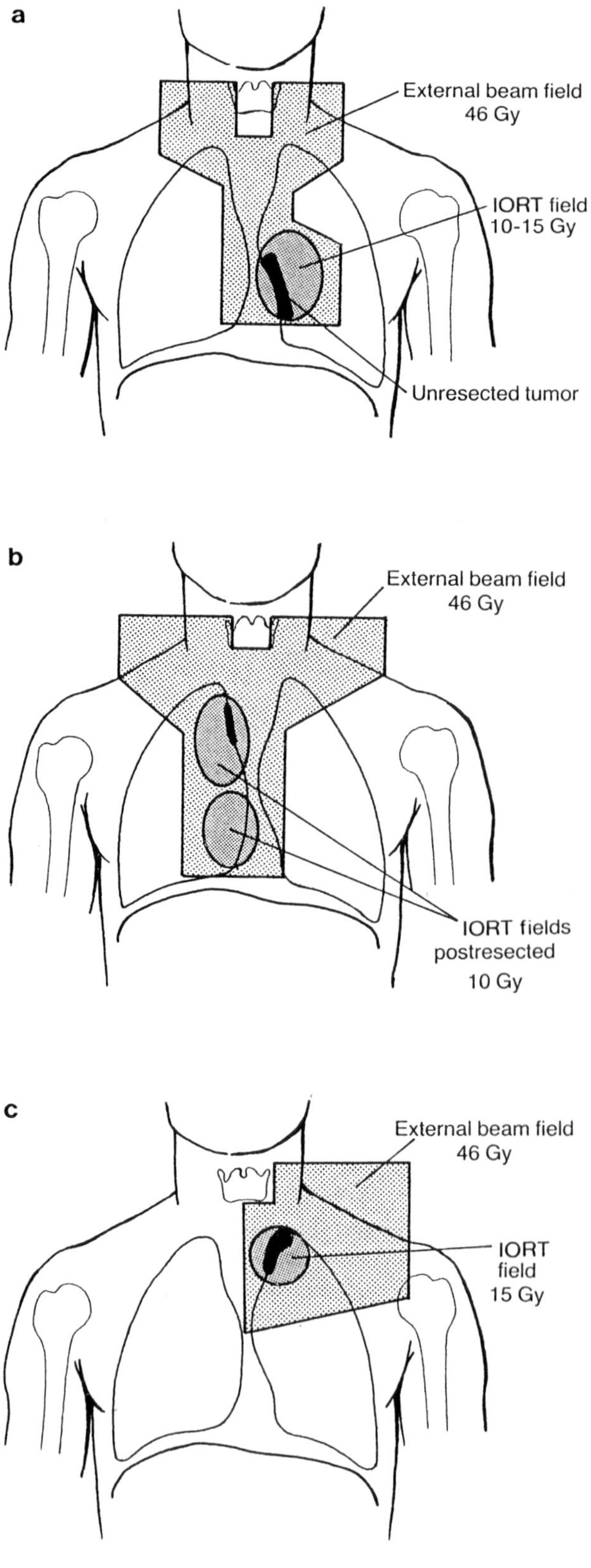

Fig. 6.1a–c. Diagram showing the integration of IORT and external beam fields

Following unilateral pneumonectomy the tolerance of mediastinal structures to 20, 25, and 30 Gy IORT (10 MeV) was analyzed. The bronchial stump healed in all dogs. Severe tissue damage was seen at all doses and included bronchovascular and esophagoaortic fistulas and esophageal stenosis (DE BOER et al. 1989).

In a different study, normal healing of the bronchial stump was found after pneumonectomy and IORT doses of 20, 30, and 40 Gy, but there were late changes with tracheobronchial radiation at all doses (5–10 months after treatment). Two out of four dogs receiving 20 Gy developed an esophageal ulcer at 6 months without late stricture. In dogs given 30 and 40 Gy esophageal damage was severe (esophagoaortic fistula and stricture) and one dog developed carinal necrosis (PASS et al. 1987).

There is a consensus among these reports that 20 Gy is the upper limit of IORT dose that can be researched in human phase I–II trials. There is no reported information on the tolerance of mediastinal and thoracic viscera to lower IORT doses (10–15 Gy) used as a boost in combination with fractionated external beam radiotherapy.

6.2.2 Clinical Results

The initial Japanese experience argued against the use of IORT in lung cancer patients owing to the early systemic dissemination observed (ABE and TAKAHASI 1981). The technique was explored in bronchogenic carcinoma during the 1970s (ABE et al. 1977). More recently, a limited phase I clinical trial indicated considerable toxicity with IORT when 25 Gy was delivered to the mediastinum following pneumonectomy (PASS et al. 1987). Of the four patients reported, three had early complications (one case of bronchial stump dehiscence, one bronchopleural fistula, and one case of reversible esophagitis), and three had late complications (one case of irreversible radiation esophagitis, one contralateral esophagobronchial fistula, and one case of reversible esophagitis). Only one patient is surviving 18 months after IORT. The protocol called for the use of two IORT fields to cover the target volume, and in one toxic case overlapping of the fields was retrospectively detected. This study recognized the feasibility of IORT during lung cancer surgery, and recommended a decrease in the IORT dose to 15–20 Gy. In unresectable tumors a European group has reported an 84% objective response rate (complete response in 4 out of 12 evaluable patients) after tumor exposure to IORT (10–20 Gy) and subsequent external beam irradiation (JUETTNER et al. 1990). The same group is studying thoracic tissue changes following IORT plus external beam radiotherapy by sophisticated diagnostic imaging techniques in an effort to correlate the findings with tumor response or progression (ARIAN-SCHAD et al. 1989).

6.3 Treatment Protocol

The locoregional treatment program has combined tumor resection (if possible), IORT boost to residual or unresectable disease, and conventional external beam radiotherapy. From the onset the IORT dose employed was 10 or 15 Gy. Several chemotherapy protocols were activated during the IORT studies, and use of locoregional intensification techniques was not rejected for this reason.

6.3.1 Surgery

All patients were approached by a lateral thoracotomy. The incision site ranged from the fourth to the sixth intercostal space depending upon tumor location. Once the thoracic cavity was opened, careful tumor staging and evaluation were carried out. In general pneumonectomy was avoided, and central lesions were exposed to the IORT field. In most of these cases a second oblique field was applied to the homolateral mediastinum. Lobectomy and atypical resections were encouraged when feasible, even in cases with a tumor margin close to the bronchial stump. Mediastinal nodal sampling was performed as a rule. An important aspect of the series was the inclusion, early on in the study, of coverage of the bronchial stump with vascularized pleural or pericardial flap if this structure was included in the IORT field. Protection of normal lung by retraction from the treatment cone was easy in patients who underwent resection. In cases of unresectable lesions, the normal portion of the lung was collapsed inside the cone (pneumonectomy was performed in only one case). Protection or mobilization of the esophagus in mediastinal IORT fields was not attempted.

6.3.2 IORT

Intraoperative radiation therapy applicators were available with diameters ranging from 5 to 15 cm and a beveled distal end (0°, 15°, 30°, and 45°) to obtain maximum adaptation to the anatomic region. IORT fields should cover areas of residual disease and/or lymphatic drainage: hilum (Fig. 6.1A), mediastinum (Fig. 6.1B), or chest wall (Fig. 6.1C). The cone diameter was selected to encircle the desired volume, comprising the tumor or tumor bed plus 1 cm of normal tissue around it. The electron energy was chosen according to the required depth of radiation penetration and depended on the thickness of the tissues at risk. Dosimetry and isodose curve distribution were calculated on a CT scan model which simulates the chest incision and tumor resection when necessary. The 90% isodose curve had to encompass the presumed target volume. If two fields were needed to treat different areas at risk (chest wall and mediastinum; hilum and mediastinum), no overlapping was allowed. Contralateral thoracic structures were not protected, but lead shielding was used in some patients with left lower or hilar lesions to prevent radiation damage to the heart and spinal cord. Unresectable tumors were introduced into the distal tip of the IORT cone and the air was forced out from the normal portion of the lung (Fig. 6.2). In these cases the source–tumor distance was modified to take into account the thickness of the tumor.

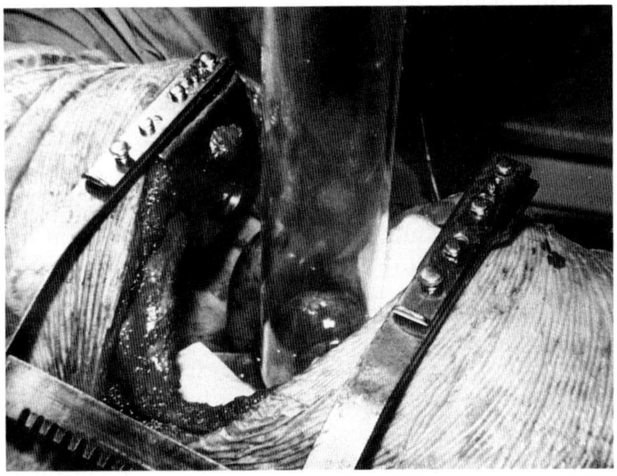

Fig. 6.2. Cone positioning for the treatment of a right hilar unresected tumor

6.3.3 External Beam Radiotherapy

In general conventional external beam radiotherapy was added 3–4 weeks after IORT. The fields were designed to cover the primary lesion (or postresection residual disease areas) and adjacent nodal areas (bilateral hilar, mediastinal, and supraclavicular). An AP-PA technique with 15 MV photons was used. Daily fractionation was 2 Gy, given 5 times per week, reaching total doses of 46–50 Gy. Preoperative external beam radiotherapy was generally selected for Pancoast lesions and tumors with chest wall involvement.

6.3.4 Chemotherapy

A group of patients analyzed proceeded to thoracotomy after three to five cycles of neoadjuvant chemotherapy with cisplatinum, mitomycin C, and vindesine (Henriquez et al. 1989).

6.4 Analysis of Results

6.4.1 General Aspects of the Series

In the early part of this program, tumor resection was not attempted in a large proportion of patients. Recently, neoadjuvant chemotherapy has allowed the tumor resection rate to be increased; during this period all patients have been clinically stage III. There were selected indications for thoracotomy in localized small cell lung cancer and these patients completed the usual treatment program for such histology (Calvo et al. 1985).

Table 6.1. Patient characteristics ($n = 60$)

	No. of patients
Age	
Median: 59 years	
Range: 35–78 years	
Sex	
Male	59
Female	1
Karnofsky performance status	
>70%	48
<70%	12
Initial symptoms	
Cough	42
Hemoptysis	22
Dyspnea	17
Superior vena cava syndrome	5
Vocal cord palsy	5
X-ray findings	2

6.4.1.1 Patient Characteristics

The total number of patients analyzed was 60; there were 59 males and one female. Their ages ranged from 35 to 78 years. Forty-eight patients (80%) had a Karnofsky performance status above 70%. Initial symptoms were cough and chest discomfort (70%). Hemoptysis and dyspnea were common. Superior vena cava compression and vocal cord palsy were present at diagnosis in a few patients (Table 6.1).

6.4.1.2 Tumor Characteristics

Squamous cell carcinoma (58%) and adenocarcinoma (23%) were the most common histologic types. Large cell, oat cell, and mixed histologies were also treated. Thirty-five tumors were located in the right hemi thorax, 21 in the left hemithorax, and four corresponded to Pancoast lesions (two on each side). Substaging showed 32 to be stage IIIa and 28, stage IIIb (Table 6.2).

6.4.1.3 Treatment Characteristics

Surgery achieved tumor resection in 43 cases, including 35 lobectomies, seven atypical lobectomies, and one pneumonectomy. A vascularized flap was used to cover the bronchial stump in 24 cases. The treatment volume was adequately encompassed by a single IORT field in 47 cases, while two IORT fields were required in 13 cases. The average cone diameter was 8 cm; 9 MeV was the most frequently used electron energy in resected lesions, as compared with 15 MeV in unresected lesions. A total of 73 nonoverlapping IORT fields were used. In 45 patients, 10 Gy was delivered in each IORT field, while in the remaining 15 patients the dose given was 15 Gy. A course of external beam radiotherapy was completed by 52 patients: 14 preoperatively and 38 postoperatively. Neoadjuvant chemotherapy was used in 22 patients eligible for a phase II study (Table 6.3).

Table 6.2. Tumor characteristics

	No. of patients
Histology	
Squamous cell	35
Adenocarcinoma	14
Large cell	2
Oat cell	3
Mixed	6
Location	
Right hemithorax	35
Hilum	6
Upper lobe	20
Middle lobe	1
Lower lobe	5
Left hemithorax	21
Hilum	8
Upper lobe	11
Lower lobe	2
Pancoast	4
Stage	
IIIa	32
IIIb	28

6.4.2 Toxicity and Complications

6.4.2.1 Tolerance of Thoracic Tissues

In patients with unresected tumors, the collapsed lung parenchyma and main bronchus (which is not surgically manipulated) were included in the

Table 6.3. Detailed treatment program characteristics

	No. of patients
Surgery	
Tumor exposure	17
Resection	43
Lobectomy	35
Atypical resection	7
Pneumonectomy	1
Use of vascularized flap	24
Pleural	22
Pericardial	2
IORT	
Cone diameter (cm)[a]	
5–7	25
8–9	34
10–12	14
Electron energy (MeV)[a]	
6–9	40
12–15	27
18–20	7
Number of fields	
Single	47
Multiple	13
Total dose (Gy)[a]	
10	45
15	15
External beam radiotherapy	
Preoperative	14
Postoperative	38
Chemotherapy	
Neoadjuvant	22
Adjuvant	6
Not given	32

[a] 73 fields treated

IORT field. Of 17 patients in this group, 14 developed acute pneumonitis in the immediate postoperative period. This was seen on the routine chest x-ray as a linear consolidation that resolved with low dose steroids (Figs. 6.3, 6.4). Of 31 patients undergoing treatment to the right mediastinum, with or without tumor resection, 18 developed transient esophagitis, generally during the later period of external beam irradiation. Esophageal stenosis did not develop in the follow-up period in any patient. Four bronchopleural fistulas were seen. One developed in the immediate postoperative period in a pneumonectomized patient, in whom the bronchial stump was not treated with IORT. In the four patients with Pancoast tumors the IORT field included the brachial plexus, and one patient developed pain and paresthesia in the ipsilateral superior extremity that disappeared over a 5-month period. As a long-term tissue change, lung fibrosis was visible on the chest x-ray in 17 cases.

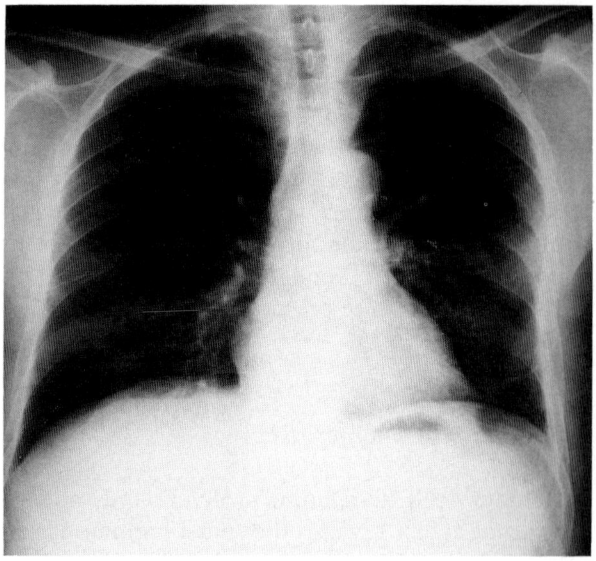

Fig. 6.4. Resolution of the x-ray findings in the patient with acute pneumonitis shown in Fig. 6.3

6.4.2.2 Patient Tolerance to the Treatment Program

There were four postoperative complications early death (pneumonia, sepsis, bronchopleural fistula, and pulmonary artery rupture, each of which occurred in one patient), leading to one and a fatal massive hemoptysis at 2 months following IORT. This latter patient had a left hilar unresected tumor, treated by tumor exposure and 15 Gy IORT plus 46 Gy external irradiation. Hemoptysis was present at diagnosis. The autopsy revealed a large necrotic cavity in the left hilum, with no viable residual tumor cells and a connection between the cavity and the hilar vascular structures (Fig. 6.5). Two patients had rib fractures at the time of surgery IORT and two others had postoperative instability of the chest wall. One patient developed a tracheoesophageal fistula, but the autopsy study revealed local tumor progression with tumor involvement of both struc-

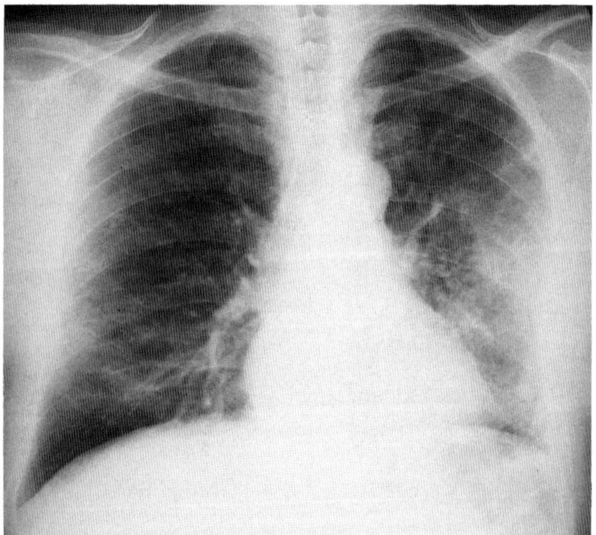

Fig. 6.3. Acute pneumonitis following IORT

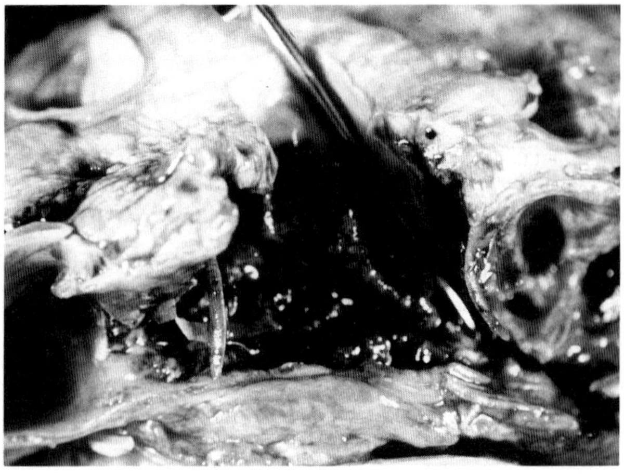

Fig. 6.5. Macroscopic autopsy findings in a patient with massive hemoptysis

Table 6.4. Tissues treated with IORT: toxicities and complications observed

Tissues treated with IORT	No. of cases
Collapsed lung parenchyma	17
Main bronchus (not manipulated)	17
Right mediastinum	31
Left mediastinum	11
Bronchial suture	33
Vascular suture	33
Chest wall	12
Brachial plexus	4
Toxicity and complications	**No. of episodes**
Postoperative period	
Pneumonia	4
Sepsis	1
Bronchopleural fistula	4
Acute pneumonitis	14
Pulmonary embolism	1
Pulmonary artery rupture	1
Short term	
Esophagitis	18
Hemoptysis	1
Instability of chest wall	2
Long term	
Neuropathy (reversible)	1
Lung fibrosis	17
Tracheoesophageal fistula	1

tures (Table 6.4). Long-term lung fibrosis was a common finding in patients surviving more than 1 year (Fig. 6.6).

6.4.3 Patterns of Relapse

Local failure is defined in this analysis as any intrathoracic tumor progression. Local failure alone as the first site of disease recurrence was seen in seven cases (six unresectable tumors, and one case with resection but with gross residual disease following surgery). Combined local and systemic progression was seen in five cases (three unresected and two resected). Distant metastasis without local progression was diagnosed in ten patients. Sites of local progression were the hilum in nine cases and the chest wall in three. Median time for local failure was 9 months, ranging from 4 to 25 months (Table 6.5). The most common sites for systemic dissemination were brain and bone. No mediastinal tumor recurrence was detected.

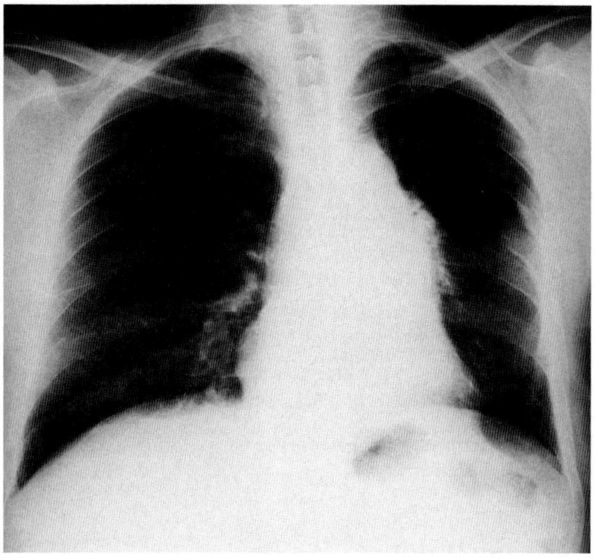

Fig. 6.6. Long-term fibrosis in a patient treated with IORT and external beam radiotherapy for an unresectable tumor; x-ray taken 12 months after treatment

6.4.4 Survival Data

At the time of this analysis 24 patients are alive and free of disease, five are alive with disease, five have died apparently free of disease, and 26 have died with disease progression. Median survival time is 12 months for the entire series. Projected actuarial survival is 28% (Fig. 6.7).

Table 6.5. Patterns of disease progression

Disease status	No. of patients	Local failure alone	Local failure+ metastasis	Distant metastasis alone
Unresectable	18	6	3	4
Resected	42	1	2	6
Gross residual disease	29	1	1	3
Microscopic residual disease	13	–	1	3
Total (%)	60 (100)	7 (11)	5 (8)	10 (16)

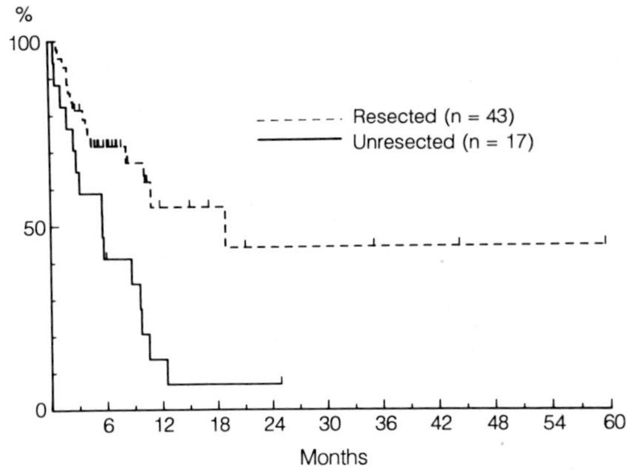

Fig. 6.7. Actuarial survival curves for patients treated with IORT for lung cancer

6.5 Conclusion

Our experience at the Clinica Universitaria de Navarra confirms the feasibility of IORT during lung cancer surgery. Tolerance of thoracic tissues to moderate doses of IORT appears to be acceptable. The use of vascularized flaps to protect the bronchial stump may prevent dehiscence of the sutures. The analysis of local recurrence suggests that thoracic disease control is related to the volume of tumor tissue treated. The local control rate in patients with tumor resection is 93%. Most thoracic recurrences were seen in the hilum (although a few patients with unresectable hilar tumors went into remission after IORT), while thoracic progression occurred in the chest wall. This supports the view that when employing IORT in lung cancer patients both central structures and the chest wall have to be considered as possible target areas. Further elucidation of the role of IORT as a locoregional intensification treatment modality in locally advanced lung cancer patients awaits further trials and the development of phase III studies. Intensive and active chemotherapy regimens have to be included in these treatment programs owing to the high rate of systemic progression of the disease.

References

Abe M, Takahashi M (1981) Intraoperative radiotherapy: the Japanese experience. Int J Radiat Oncol Biol Phys 7: 863–868

Abe M, Yabumoto E, Nishidai T, Takahashi M (1977) Trials of new forms of radiotherapy for locally advanced bronchogenic carcinoma. Strahlentherapie 153: 149–158

Arian-Schad K, Flueckinger F, Ebner F, Juettner F, Leitner H, Hackl A (1989) Treatment of primary lung cancer with combined intraoperative radiation therapy and external beam radiation: evaluation of response with CT/MRI imaging. Int J Radiat Oncol Biol Phys 17 [Suppl 1]: 222

Barnes M, Pass H, de Luca A et al. (1987) Response of the mediastinal and thoracic viscera of the dog to intraoperative radiation therapy (IORT). Int J Radiat Oncol Biol Phys 13: 371–378

Calvo FA, Harguindey SS, Anton-Aparicio L et al. (1985) Urokinase and combination chemotherapy for the treatment of small cell carcinoma of the lung. Cancer Treat Symp 2: 105–108

Calvo FA, Ortiz de Urbina D, Abuchaibe O et al. (1990) Intraoperative radiotherapy during lung cancer surgery: technical description and early clinical results. Int J Radiat Oncol Biol Phys 19: 103–109

Cox JD (1983) Failure analysis of inoperable carcinoma of the lung of all histopathologic types and squamous cell carcinoma of the esophagus. Cancer Treat Symp 2: 77–86

de Boer WJ, Mehta DM, Oosterhuis JW et al. (1989) Tolerance of mediastinal structures to intraoperative radiotherapy after pneumonectomy in dogs. Strahlenther Onkol 165: 768

Emami B, Perez CA (1987) Carcinoma of the lung. In: Perez CA, Brady LW (eds) Principles and practice of radiation oncology. JB Lippincott, Philadelphia, pp 650–683

Henriquez I, Munoz L, Ortiz de Urbina D et al. (1989) Neoadjuvant chemotherapy with cisplatin (CDDP), vindesine (VDS) and mitomycin C (MMC) in locally advanced non-small cell lung cancer (NSCLC) (abstract P-0066). Proc ECCO5, London, September 1989

Holmes EC, Gail M (1986) Lung Cancer Study Group: surgical adjuvant therapy for stage II and stage III adenocarcinoma and large-cell undifferentiated carcinoma. J Clin Oncol 4: 710–715

Juettner FM, Arian-Schad K, Porsch G et al. (1990) Intraoperative megavolt radiation therapy combined with external radiation in nonresectable non-small cell lung cancer: preliminary report. Int J Radiat Oncol Biol Phys 18: 1143–1150

Litcher AS, Bunn PA, Ihde DC et al. (1985) The role of radiation therapy in the treatment of small cell lung cancer. Cancer 55: 2163–2175

Martini N, Kris MG, Gralla RJ et al. (1987) The effects of preoperative chemotherapy on the resectability of non-small cell lung carcinoma with mediastinal lymph node metastasis (N2 M0) (abstract). Proc Soc Thor Surg 23: 28

Pass HI, Sindelar WF, Kinsella TJ et al. (1987) Delivery of intraoperative radiation therapy after pneumonectomy: experimental observations and early clinical results. Ann Thorac Surg 44: 14–20

Richards F, Scarantino CW (1985) Results of clinical trials and basis for future therapeutics. In: Scarantino CW (ed) Lung cancer. Springer, Berlin Heildelberg New York, pp 97–126

7 Gastric Cancer

FELIPE A. CALVO, MANUEL SANTOS, FERNANDO PARDO, JOSÉ L. HERNÁNDEZ, JAVIER ALVAREZ-CIENFUEGOS, and JUAN VOLTAS

CONTENTS

7.1 Introduction 51
7.2 Previous Experiences 51
7.2.1 Tissue Tolerance Studies 51
7.2.2 Clinical Results 52
7.3 Treatment Protocol 52
7.4 Results 54
7.4.1 Patient, Tumor, and Treatment Characteristics 54
7.4.2 Toxicity and Complications 54
7.4.3 Outcome: Follow-up Data 54
7.5 Conclusion 55
References 56

7.1 Introduction

Gastric cancer is the disease for which the most interesting and attractive data have been produced using IORT. The pioneering work of Dr. ABE in developing this treatment modality is particularly evident in the gastric cancer trial performed at the University of Kyoto (ABE 1984).

The use of locoregional intensification treatment programs in localized gastric cancer is supported by careful analysis of the behavior of this disease. The patterns of recurrence of resected gastric cancer have shown a tendency for initial progression to occur in locoregional structures (GUNDERSON 1987). Following curative resection, locoregional recurrences as the first and only form of disease progression were found in 22% of cases, while in 67% there was a combination of locoregional recurrence and disease in distant areas (GUNDERSON and SOSIN 1982). However, the presumed poor tolerance to high dose external beam radiotherapy of some of the structures and organs contained in the upper abdomen has limited the interest in including this modality in clinical trials of adjuvant therapy in gastric cancer. Early studies reported a 7%–20% long-term survival rate in patients treated with radiotherapy following noncurative resection (ASAKAWA and TAKEDA 1973; FALKSON and FALKSON 1969; MORTEL et al. 1969). In the past decade there has been renewed interest in exploring radiotherapy in the management of gastric cancer; this has taken the form of either external beam irradiation in combination with surgery and chemotherapy (GEZ et al. 1986; SINDELAR et al. 1986) or IORT boost with postoperative external beam radiotherapy (CALVO and HANKS 1988).

FELIPE A. CALVO, Director and Consultant, MANUEL SANTOS, Dr., Radiotherapy Division, FERNANDO PARDO, Dr., Consultant, JOSÉ L. HERNÁNDEZ Dr., Consultant, JAVIER ALVAREZ-CIENFUEGOS, Dr., Consultant, JUAN VOLTAS; Dr., Consultant, Department of Surgery, Clinica Universitaria de Navarra, 31080 Pamplona, Spain

7.2 Previous Experiences

7.2.1 Tissue Tolerance Studies

Following gastrectomy the target volume for IORT comprises the central abdominal nodes located in the celiac axis and the tumor bed in patients with medial or proximal primary tumors. The normal tissues included in the field will be the aorta, the celiac trunk, vertebral bodies, the pancreas, and the sutured left gastric artery. Animal studies have shown minor histologic changes in large vessels treated with IORT doses below 20 Gy, either alone (KINSELLA and SINDELAR 1985) or in combination with external beam radiotherapy (50 Gy) (GILLETTE et al. 1989). Pancreatic fibrosis with atrophy and exocrine pancreatic insufficiency has been described in dogs treated with IORT plus external beam irradiation. A dose–response relationship was observed for the incidence of late pancreatic damage. Exocrine pancreatic insufficiency developed in one dog treated with 25 Gy IORT and 50 Gy external beam irradiation (AHMADU-SUKA et al. 1988).

A variety of complications have been reported in clinical trials using IORT in gastric cancer, with or without external beam radiotherapy. The largest Japanese series described slight increases in serum insulin and amylase values in the immediate postoperative period following IORT doses of 20–30 Gy; the serum levels decreased to normal values in the follow-up period (Abe 1984). Further complications have been reported from the same institution: one case of ulceration of the remnant stomach which penetrated the abdominal aorta (1.5 years after IORT) and two cases of common bile duct stricture (1 and 2.5 years after IORT) requiring surgical repair (Honda et al. 1988). Other groups have reported complications in IORT gastric trials including gastrointestinal bleeding, vascular complications, and infections (Maher et al. 1988). In our own series, pancreatic fistula, vertebral collapse, and development of liver hemangiomas were initially observed as treatment-related IORT complications (Calvo et al. 1989).

7.2.2 Clinical Results

The data regarding gastric IORT produced at the University of Kyoto have been continually updated (Abe and Takahashi 1981; Abe 1984; Takahashi and Abe 1986). To summarize, the study compared surgery alone with surgery plus single dose 18–40 Gy IORT in resectable gastric cancer. The IORT field encompassed the areas of residual tumor of the celiac axis nodes. Pentagonal IORT cones of different sizes were used to define the treatment zone. The survival figures after 5 years were as follows: stage I, 93% surgery alone (43 patients treated) vs 87% surgery plus IORT (24); stage II, 61% surgery alone (11) vs 83% surgery plus IORT (20); stage III, 36% surgery alone (38) vs 62% surgery plus IORT (30); stage IV, 0% surgery alone (18) vs 14% surgery plus IORT (27) (Abe 1989). This expert group has recommended the integration of IORT into the management of gastric cancer (Abe et al. 1989).

Results have also been reported from a randomized study carried out at the National Cancer Institute (USA). The study design selected patients with stage III and IV tumors that were grossly resected. The treatment arms compared gastrectomy plus 20 Gy IORT (11 MeV) or 50 Gy external beam radiotherapy. Ten patients received IORT while 18 were treated with external beam irradiation. Actuarial survival in the IORT group was 20 months, which was superior to the 10.2 months survival in the external irradiation group (difference not statistically significant). The median disease-free interval for the IORT patients was 14.2 months, compared with 6.9 months for those who received external beam irradiation. Local disease control was prolonged in the IORT group (median time to local failure, 10.8 months) as compared with the external beam irradiation group (8.0 months). The authors concluded that IORT enhances local control compared with conventional therapy, and does not increase the incidence of treatment complications (Sindelar and Kinsella 1987).

Further experience is available from another Japanese institution. In a 4-year period, 43 patients with gastric cancer were treated with IORT (20–30 Gy): 19 following curative resection, 21 with residual disease after operation, and three with unresected tumors. The 4-year survival rates were 80%, 6%, and 0%, respectively (Ogata et al. 1988).

7.3 Treatment Protocol

In our institution the surgical approach to the upper abdomen was in the past made through various types of incision: median xiphopubic, bilateral subtotal laparotomy, etc. In 1986 the surgical approach was modified; since then we have used a transverse incision with a lower concavity, the center of which passes approximately 3 cm from the umbilicus. After the abdominal cavity has been explored and the treatment decision taken, another medial incision is made from the xiphoid, down midline to the main transverse incision. The two remaining upper flaps of skin are raised to ensure their preservation and are temporarily sutured at the hypogastric level. Thus, a wide exposure of the upper and median abdominal cavity is achieved, allowing an easy surgical technique and proper positioning of the IORT cones.

During the IORT procedure, the patient lies in a supine position. The IORT cones used for gastric carcinomas are always beveled (15°–30°) and the gantry of the linear accelerator is angulated to allow a better location of the cone under the ribs and sternum. The type of surgical incision described has been found to be very helpful for positioning of the IORT cone. The anatomic space open in the upper abdomen facilitates the movement of the esophagojejunal suture, the transverse colon, and other mobile structures of the upper abdomen, such as the small bowel. The fixed part of the duodenum is not included in the IORT field. The liver is pushed up with a retractor. Following gastrectomy, the patient is transported to the room containing the linear accelerator. Once the surgical area is exposed again, the appropriate IORT cone is selected and positioned to cover the lymph node areas of the celiac axis, the upper two-thirds of the head and body of the pancreas, and the medial portions of the hepatic and splenic hilum. The remaining intra-abdominal structures (duodenum, liver, transverse colon, small bowel, and esophageal infradiaphragmatic portion) are mobilized and protected from the radiation field (Fig. 7.1). Circular treatment cones ranging from 6 to 10 cm in diameter, with bevel angles ranging from 15° to 30°, are used. The total dose delivered ranges from 10 to 20 Gy, 15 Gy being the dose most commonly used. The selected electron beam energy ranges from 9 to 20 MeV. The dose is prescribed to the 90% isodose curve. Once the procedure is completed, the patient is transported back to the operating room, where the surgical procedure is finished.

The external beam irradiation technique consists of the treatment of a volume covering the lymph nodes contained in the upper abdomen, including the celiac axis, para-aortic, peripancreatic, and gastric bed area. Parallel opposed fields (AP-PA) of 15 MV photons are used; both fields are treated every day with custom-designed shielding blocks. Daily fractionation is 1.8–2 Gy, 5 times per week, reaching a total dose of 46 Gy. The treatment was started 4 weeks after the surgical procedure (Fig. 7.2). The estimated total dose delivered to the spinal cord in this treatment program depends upon two components: the dose received from the IORT, and the dose given during fractionated external beam irradiation. The IORT component has been calculated with body tomography simulations. For 9–12 MeV electron beams, the estimated isodose reaching the spinal cord ranges from 2% to 9%. In cases with higher electron beam energies (15–20 MeV), this estimation is still valid because of the amount of residual tumor tissue left following gastrectomy. The external beam radiotherapy program has been performed with 15 MV photons in all cases, using parallel opposed fields, and the spinal cord lies on the 102% isodose curve. Combining the information, it can be estimated that the total dose received by the spinal cord does not exceed 50 Gy

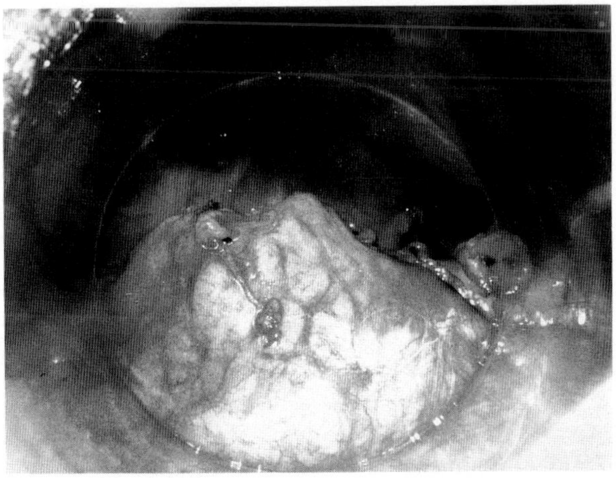

Fig. 7.1. View of the treatment field through the IORT cone following resection of gastric cancer

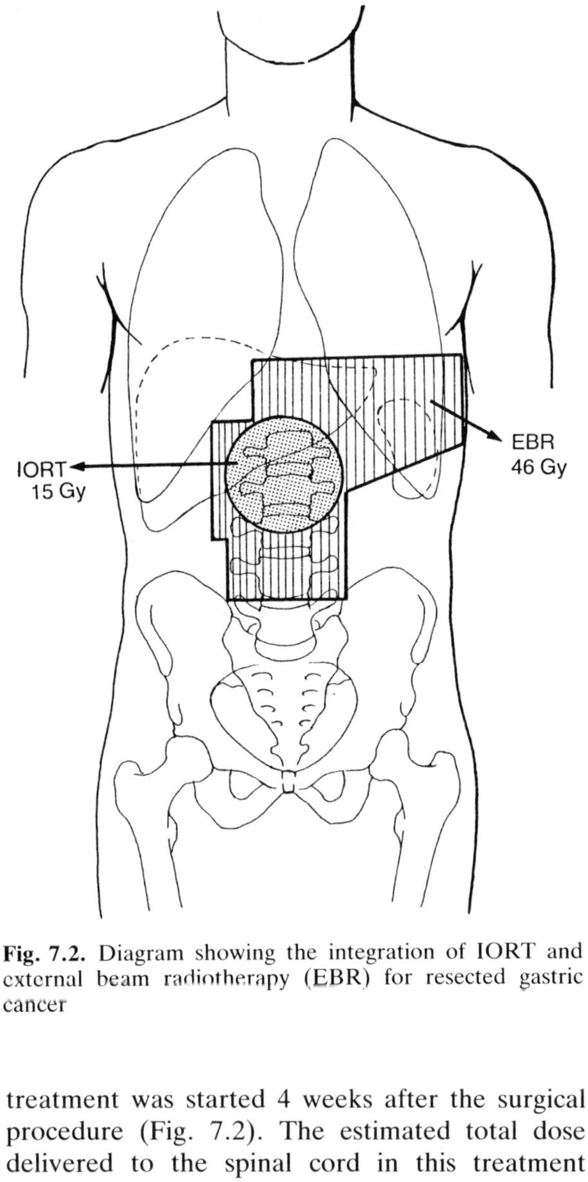

Fig. 7.2. Diagram showing the integration of IORT and external beam radiotherapy (EBR) for resected gastric cancer

in 10 weeks (the total duration of the radiotherapy treatment program). A previous report from our group described in detail many technical aspects of the treatment program (Calvo et al. 1989).

7.4 Results

7.4.1 Patient, Tumor, and Treatment Characteristics

Between September 1984 and October 1989, a total of 48 patients with gastric neoplasms were treated with surgery and IORT. For the purpose of this study, 43 patients were analyzed. Of the five patients excluded, three had a different histologic diagnosis (lymphomas and sarcoma) and two were lost to follow-up soon after treatment. The patients ranged in age from 34 to 82 years (median 62 years); there were 32 males and 11 females. Karnofsky performance status was above 70% in 26 patients. Initial symptoms at the time of diagnosis of gastric cancer included weight loss, anemia, gastrointestinal bleeding, dysphagia, and nausea and vomiting. In four cases the tumor had recurred at the stump of a previous gastrectomy. All patients had adenocarcinoma; 15 cases were moderately to well differentiated while 28 were diffuse and/or undifferentiated. Tumor location was peripyloric or distal in 24 cases and central in nine. Postsurgical staging showed 27 cases to be stage III, nine stage IV, and seven stage I–II. Total gastrectomy was performed in 35 cases, partial gastrectomy in one, and exposure of nodal sites of recurrence in the celiac axis area in two. The IORT cone size was 7 or more centimeters in diameter in 37 procedures. The electron energy most commonly used was 12 MeV. The total single dose delivered to the IORT volume was 15 Gy in 41 cases. External beam radiotherapy was omitted in five stage I–II cases. In nine patients with diffuse undifferentiated histology, adjuvant chemotherapy (continuous infusion of cisplatin plus 5-fluorouracil for 5 days, repeated every 4 weeks for six courses) was added to the treatment program (Table 7.1).

Table 7.1. Tumor and treatment characteristics in patients treated with IORT for resectable gastric cancer

	No. of patients
Tumor	
Histology (adenocarcinoma)	43
Moderately/well differentiated	15
Diffuse/undifferentiated	28
Location	
Proximal	6
Central	9
Distal	24
Stump recurrence	4
Stage	
I-II	7
III	27
IV	9
Treatment	
Surgery	
Total gastrectomy	35
Partial gastrectomy	1
Tumor exposure	2
IORT dose (Gy)	
10	1
15	41
20	1
Cone diameter (cm)	
5–6	6
7–8	20
9–10	17
Number of fields	
Single	43
Multiple	–
Electron energy (Mev)	
6–9	13
12–15	27
18–20	3
External irradiation	
Preoperative	2
Postoperative	36
Not done	5
Chemotherapy	
Yes	9
No	34

7.4.2 Toxicity and Complications

A careful analysis has been made of all medical problems observed in patients treated with this protocol. There were 25 episodes of acute postoperative complications, seen in 15 patients (35%). These findings included nausea and vomiting, pneumonia, dumping syndrome, diarrhea, pleural effusion, suture dehiscence, pulmonary abscess, cholangitis, and esophageal hemorrhage. In the follow-up period, 11 medical problems were encountered in ten (23%) patients; they included vertebral collapse, liver hemangioma, dysphagia, liver infarction, and bleeding from an aneurysm which developed from the stump of the left gastric artery (Table 7.2).

7.4.3 Outcome: Follow-up Data

At the time of this analysis ten patients have died with progressive malignant disease. Five had stage

Table 7.2. Toxicity and complications in patients treated with IORT for resectable gastric cancer

	No. of patients	No. of episodes
Acute	15 (35%)	25 (69%)
Nausea/vomiting		5 (14%)
Pneumonia		5 (14%)
Dumping syndrome		5 (14%)
Diarrhea		3 (8%)
Pleural effusion		2 (6%)
Suture dehiscence		2 (6%)
Abdominal-pulmonary abscess[a]		1 (3%)
Cholangitis[a]		1 (3%)
Esophageal hemorrhage[a]		1 (3%)
Late	10 (23%)	11 (31%)
Vertebral collapse		3 (8%)
Liver hemangioma		3 (8%)
Dysphagia		2 (6%)
Hemochromatosis		1 (3%)
Liver infarction[a]		1 (3%)
Celiac aneurysm[a]		1 (3%)

[a] Life-threatening complications (5%–13%; IORT associated, 2%–5%)

IV or recurrent disease and five, stage III disease. The sites of first failure were upper abdominal (liver, hepatic portal, and/or celiac axis) in all except one patient with lung metastases. Histologic subtype was diffuse undifferentiated in eight and well differentiated in two (Tables 7.3, 7.4). The follow-up time ranges from 2+ to 52+ months. The actuarial survival curve for the entire group is shown in Fig. 7.3. A separate analysis has evaluated survival as a function of postsurgical disease status (macroscopic vs microscopic residual disease) (Fig. 7.4).

Table 7.3. Treatment failure in relation to treatment parameters

Treatment parameters	Site of progression					No. of patients
	Intra-abdominal			Extra-abdominal		
	CA	P	Li	B	Lu	
Cone diameter (cm)						
6	1		4	1		4
7					1	1
8		2				2
9	1	1		1		2
10	1					1
Electron energy (Mev)						
9	1	1		1	1	3
12		1	2	1		4
15		1				1
18	1		1			1
20	1		1			1
No. of patients	3	3	4	2	1	10

Abbreviations: CA, celiac axis; P, peritoneum; Li, liver; B, bone; Lu, lung

Table 7.4. Treatment failure in relation to tumor characteristics

Tumor characteristics	Site of progression					No. of patients
	Intra-abdominal			Extra-abdominal		
	CA	P	Li	B	Lu	
Stage						
III	1	2		1	1	4
IV	2	1	4	1		6
Residual disease						
Macroscopic	2	2	4	1	1	8
Microscopic	1	1		1		2
Histology						
Well differentiated	1		1		1	2
Undifferentiated	2	3	3	2		8
No. of patients	3	3	4	2	1	10

Abbreviations: CA, celiac axis; P, peritoneum; Li, liver; B, bone; Lu, lung

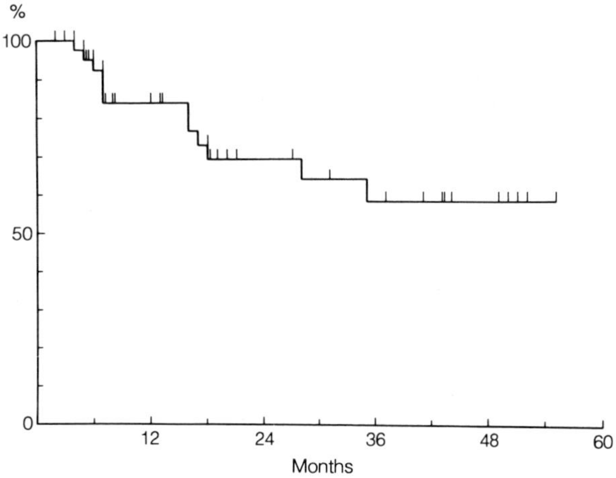

Fig. 7.3. Actuarial survival curve for the entire group of gastric cancer patients treated with gastrectomy, IORT, and external beam radiotherapy

7.5 Conclusion

It is feasible to integrate IORT into a combined approach for resectable gastric cancer. The protocol explored, which used moderate doses of IORT (15 Gy) and external beam radiotherapy, appears to be tolerated, but is at the upper limit of acceptable therapy intensity. Although long-term results are not yet available, the initial data regarding projected survival in locally advanced and intermediate tumor stages are encouraging.

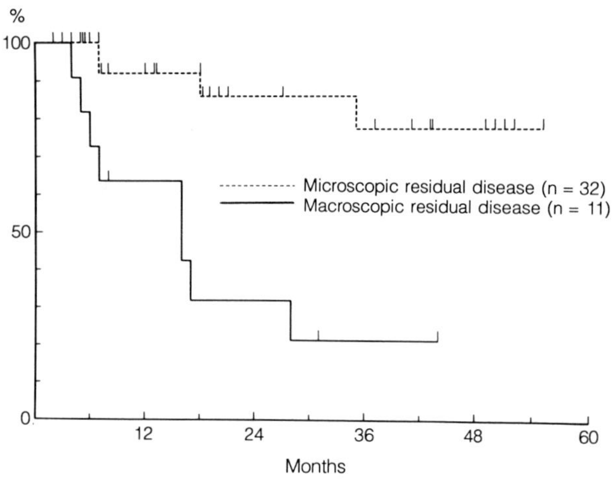

Fig. 7.4. Actuarial survival curves in patients with microscopic or macroscopic residual disease following surgery

References

Abe M (1984) Intraoperative radiation therapy for gastrointestinal malignancy. In: De Cosse JJ, Sherlock P (eds) Clinical management of gastrointestinal cancer. Martinus Nijhoff, New York, pp 327–349

Abe M (1989) Intraoperative radiation therapy for gastric cancer. In: Dobelbower RR, Abe M (eds) Intraoperative radiation therapy. CRC, Boca Raton, Fl, pp 165–180

Abe M, Takahashi M (1981) Intraoperative radiotherapy: the Japanese experience. Int J Radiat Oncol Biol Phys 7:863–868

Abe M, Takahashi M, Ono K et al. (1989) Japanese gastric trials in intraoperative radiation therapy. Int J Radiat Oncol Biol Phys 15:1431–1433

Ahmadu-Suka F, Gillete EL, Vithrow SJ et al. (1988) Pathologic response of the pancreas and duodenum to experimental intraoperative irradiation. Int J Radiat Oncol Biol Phys 14:1197–1204

Asakawa H, Takeda T (1973) High energy x-ray therapy of gastric carcinoma. J Jpn Soc Cancer Ther 8:362–371

Calvo FA, Hanks GE (1988) Intraoperative trials. Int J Radiat Oncol Biol Phys 14:S111–S117

Calvo FA, Henriquez I, Santos M et al. (1989) Intraoperative and external beam radiotherapy in advanced resectable gastric cancer: technical description and preliminary results. Int J Radiat Oncol Biol Phys 17:183–189

Falkson G, Falkson C (1969) Fluorouracil and radiotherapy in gastric cancer. Lancet 2:1252–1253

Gez E, Sielkes A, Yablonsky PT (1986) Combined 5-FU and radiation therapy following resection of locally advanced gastric carcinoma. J Surg Oncol 31:139–142

Gillette EL, Powers BE, McChesney SL et al. (1989) Response of aorta and branch arteries to experimental intraoperative irradiation. Int J Radiat Oncol Biol Phys 17:1247–1255

Gunderson LL (1987) Gastric cancer. In: Perez CA, Brady LW (eds) Principles and practice of radiation oncology. JB Lippincott, Philadelphia, pp 793–800

Gunderson LL, Sosin H (1982) Adenocarcinoma of the stomach: areas of failure in a reoperation series (second or symptomatic looks): clinico-pathologic correlation and implications for adjuvant therapy. Int J Radiat Oncol Biol Phys 8:1–11

Honda K, Inamoto T, Shibamoto Y et al. (1988) Intraoperative radiation therapy for gastric cancer. Strahlenther Onkol 165:776

Kinsella TJ, Sindelar WF (1985) Intraoperative radiotherapy. In: De Vita VT, Hellman S, Rosenberg SA, (eds) Principles and practice of oncology. JB Lippincott, Philadelphia, pp 2293–2304

Maher MM, Cromack DA, White DE et al. (1988) Complications of intraoperative radiation therapy. Strahlenther Onkol 165:783

Moertel CG, Chilos DS, Retitemeier RJ et al. (1969) Combined 5-fluorouracil and supervoltage radiation of unresectable gastrointestinal cancer. Lancet II:865–867

Ogata T, Yamashita AK, Sugimoto MT et al. (1988) Combined surgical and intraoperative radiation therapy of the cancer of the digestive organs. Strahlenther Onkol 165:773

Sindelar WF, Kinsella TJ (1987) Randomized trial of resection and intraoperative radiotherapy in locally advanced gastric cancer. Proc Am Soc Clin Oncol 6:91

Sindelar WF, Hoekstra H, Restrepo C et al. (1986) Pathological tissue changes following intraoperative radiotherapy. Am J Clin Oncol 9:504–509

Takahashi M, Abe M (1986) Intra-operative radiotherapy for carcinoma of the stomach. Eur J Surg Oncol 12: 247–250

8 Pancreatic Cancer

FELIPE A. CALVO, IGNACIO AZINOVIC, GERARDO ZORNOZA,
JUAN VOLTAS, FERNANDO PARDO, and JAVIER ALVAREZ-CIENFUEGOS

CONTENTS

8.1 Introduction ... 57
8.2 Previous Experiences ... 57
8.2.1 Tissue Tolerance Studies ... 57
8.2.2 Clinical Results ... 58
8.3 Treatment Protocol ... 60
8.4 Results ... 60
8.4.1 General Aspects of the Series ... 60
8.4.2 Toxicity and Complications ... 61
8.4.3 Patterns of Relapse ... 61
8.4.4 Survival ... 62
8.5 Conclusion ... 62
References ... 62

8.1 Introduction

The pancreas is the disease site most frequently treated with IORT (DOBELBOWER and ABE 1989). This tumor location can benefit from the advantages of IORT: the tumor is accurately defined at the time of surgery and the surrounding normal tissues can be mobilized to expose the tumor to the electron beam. These positive aspects have led to high expectations regarding the results of intensive locoregional treatment including IORT. On the other hand, it is well known that cancer of the pancreas is rarely a resectable tumor at the time of diagnosis, and even in patients who undergo resection, long-term survival rates are modest. In general, patients with pancreatic cancer will be surgically evaluated to determine resectability; if the lesion is not considered for radical surgery then a biopsy, to confirm malignancy, and a biliary and gastrointestinal bypass are performed. The median survival time for patients with locally advanced disease treated with palliative surgery is 6–8 months, while for those with disseminated disease it is 2–4 months. Following radical surgery the median survival time is 12 months, with a 10%–20% long-term survival rate (SINDELAR et al. 1985a).

Intraoperative radiation therapy is a treatment modality that allows one to deliver radical doses of radiation in cases of unresectable and resected pancreatic cancer, particularly if external beam radiotherapy is included in the treatment program. This approach might promote local tumor control, but an ultimate benefit in survival may not result if there is a high rate of distant dissemination of the disease. In fact, at the present time, and with the information available, clinical trials using IORT for the treatment of carcinoma of the pancreas have yielded results that are of some interest for the management of this disease site but do not represent a major step forward in terms of survival. Among the positive findings that are constantly reported in IORT trials are: an excellent palliative effect for abdominal pain as a tumor-associated symptom (WILLICH et al. 1989a); a median survival time in the range of 9–12 months for patients with localized unresectable lesions (GUNDERSON et al. 1987; ROLDAN et al. 1988); and local tumor control promotion, particularly in cases that have undergone resection (SINDELAR and KINSELLA 1986a). The combination of IORT as a boosting modality with fractionated external beam irradiation seems to increase slightly the median survival time when compared with IORT alone (MATSUDA and TANAKA 1989).

8.2 Previous Experiences

8.2.1 Tissue Tolerance Studies

In the case of unresectable pancreatic cancer the tissues to be included in the IORT field are: the

FELIPE A. CALVO, Dr., Director and Consultant, IGNACIO AZINOVIC, Dr., Radiotherapy Division, Department of Oncology, GERARDO ZORNOZA, Dr., Consultant, JUAN VOLTAS, Dr., Consultant, FERNANDO PARDO, Dr., Consultant, JAVIER ALVAREZ-CIENFUEGOS, Dr., Consultant, Department of Surgery, Clinica Universitaria de Navarra, 31080 Pamplona, Spain tumor mass, normal pancreatic parenchyma, the vessels of the celiac trunk, the inferior vena cava, the aorta, and vertebral bodies posteriorly. In addition these structures sometimes have to be partially included in the IORT field in the case of resectable tumors located in the head of the pancreas or extending inferiorly to the C-loop of the duodenum (which can be either involved by the lesion or too close to it).

In most instances the common bile duct will be included as well, either because it is already stenotic in an intratumoral portion or due to the normal tissue margin that is always sought in the selection of the IORT cone size. Other organs and structures of the upper abdomen, such as the stomach, transverse colon, and small bowel, can be easily mobilized during the surgical procedure. Sometimes the surgeon is tempted to expose the tumor through the upper or small curvature of the stomach, pulling down this organ. In general this has the disadvantage that the treatment field is poorly visualized and careful palpation will show tumor extension inferiorly, further away than the limits of exposure achieved by pulling down the stomach. In addition the stomach can slip into the IORT field during the IORT procedure if the cone is not firmly fixed.

Animal studies have prospectively analyzed the tolerance of several of these upper abdominal structures to a high single dose of IORT, with or without fractionated external beam irradiation.

Clinical data on normal tissue changes following IORT in patients with a variety of tumors have been reported by the National Cancer Institute (USA) investigators (Sindelar et al. 1986). In a further analysis by the same group, the histologic changes observed in patients with carcinoma of the pancreas were described (Hoekstra et al. 1988). Among 33 patients treated, 13 underwent autopsy with careful examination of the tissues included in the IORT field. Six of the 13 died in the postoperative period, with a follow-up ranging from 2 to 7 weeks after IORT. In the remaining seven patients the follow-up ranged from 3 to 18 months; all died from metastatic disease except for one patient who developed late nutritional deficiency and bronchopneumonia while free of neoplastic disease. In three patients external beam radiotherapy was added to 20–27.5 Gy IORT electrons. Moderate to severe radiation effects were observed in all patients treated for unresectable pancreatic cancer. These effects consisted in pancreatic fibrosis, vascular sclerosis, nerve degeneration, atrophy of acinar cells, and atypical epithelial changes in the ducts. Islands of viable tumor cells were always present. Retroperitoneal and porta hepatis fibrosis were late macroscopic and microscopic findings in long-term survivors. The aorta and vena cava did not show histologic changes, but the superior mesenteric artery displayed subintimal fibrosis in six of nine patients who had undergone a total pancreatectomy. The vertebral bodies showed focal marrow hypocellularity in six patients with pancreatic resection. In addition there were various other findings in this study which could not easily be correlated with radiation effects, i.e., hepatic steatosis, cholestasis, biliary cirrhosis, and hepatic necrosis. In none of the eight patients with such liver or bile duct changes were these structures included in the irradiated field.

Several toxicities and complications in surrounding normal tissues have been described in clinical reports: rupture of the superior mesenteric artery, duodenal and gastric ulcers, stricture of the common bile duct (Goldson et al. 1981), pancreatic insufficiency (Tepper et al. 1987), and gastrointestinal bleeding from radiation duodenitis (Sindelar et al. 1985b).

In summary, normal tissues and structures of the upper abdomen might limit the tolerance to IORT for carcinoma of the pancreas. The duodenum, bile duct, superior mesenteric artery, and normal pancreas are fixed structures that have to be included in the IORT field and may show long-term changes. Biliary and gastrointestinal bypass has been recommended to minimize long-term effects in patients with unresectable pancreatic tumors (Hoekstra et al. 1988). There is a lack of information regarding the clinical importance of retroperitoneal fibrosis, bone marrow hypocellularity, and tolerance of vascular sutures in patients treated with IORT following pancreatic resection. If this modality is used in an adjuvant fashion (Heijmans et al. 1989), these structures would be the clinically important normal tissues at risk for radiation damage.

8.2.2 Clinical Results

In the last decade, numerous institutions and research groups have reported their experience in the treatment of pancreatic cancer with IORT. Apart from the fact that scientific literature is concentrated on this disease site in both Japan

(Abe and Takahashi 1981; Nishimura et al. 1984; Hiraoka et al. 1984; Abe et al. 1987; Yasue 1988; Kamata et al. 1989; Hata et al. 1989; Kita et al. 1989; Nakano et al. 1989; Tanaka et al. 1989) and the United States (Goldson et al. 1981; Wood et al. 1982; Shipley et al. 1984; Sindelar and Kinsela 1986a,b; Gunderson et al. 1987), the emerging European studies also focus particularly on the pancreas (Bodner et al. 1986; Huguier et al. 1987; Calvo et al. 1987; Hoekstra et al. 1989; Glaser et al. 1989; Dubois 1989; Willich et al. 1988, 1989a,b; Bodner and Glaser 1989). In an effort to highlight the relevant points of interest that have emerged regarding the use of IORT in the management of pancreatic cancer, some particular topics have been selected for discussion here.

At the present time IORT is recognized as a sophisticated radiation boosting modality which it is feasible to integrate in the multidisciplinary management of resectable and unresectable pancreatic cancer. Some technical limitations have been found when dealing with fixed structures (duodenum, bile duct, superior mesenteric artery), necessitating individualized consideration of palliative surgical maneuvers (bypasses) and adequate IORT technique (field size, electron energy, etc.). Survival data include two parameters of particular interest: median survival time and long-term survival rate.

The median survival times reported vary widely, from 4.5 to 17 months, although most studies in the second half of the 1980s have reported values between 8 and 10 months. It appears that the differences are related to patient selection criteria, tumor staging systems, and variations in treatment protocol. On the other hand, a common finding in all studies is that few, if any, long-term survivors are seen. Several reports have analyzed particular aspects of interest, such as the local tumor control rates compared with those obtained with high dose external beam radiotherapy alone, and the simultaneous use of hypoxic cell sensitizers or hyperthermia. At the Mayo Clinic, 3 out of 42 (7%) evaluable patients developed local progression following 45–50 Gy external beam radiotherapy and 17.5–20 Gy IORT boost (Gunderson et al. 1987). The same group compared the results obtained in their institution in patients with unresectable pancreatic cancer treated by either external beam radiotherapy alone (40–60 Gy, 122 patients) or external irradiation plus an IORT boost (45–55 Gy, 37 patients). Most patients received chemotherapy with 5-fluorouracil. The local control rates at 1 year were 48% and 83% and at 2 years, 20% and 66%, respectively ($P < 0.0005$). Differences in median or long-term survival of the two treatment groups were not statistically significant (median 12.6 months vs 13.4 months) (Roldan et al. 1988). Radiation response modifiers such as misonidazole (Tepper et al. 1987) and hyperthermia (Goldson et al. 1989; Merrik et al. 1989) have been studied in conjunction with IORT in an attempt to increase further local control rates in unresectable cancer of the pancreas.

At the National Cancer Institute (USA) two randomized clinical trials have investigated the possible role of IORT in carcinoma of the pancreas. Both studies included 32 patients, half of whom were randomly selected to receive IORT boost. One study concerned resectable disease, and one, unresectable disease; in the former case no external beam irradiation was given.

Operative mortality was high (9 out of 32 patients) in the study with pancreatic resection and IORT boost. Median survival time was similar in the IORT and the control groups (12 months). The disease-free interval was longer in IORT patients (20 months) than in controls (12 months) when operative deaths were excluded from the analysis. The local disease control rate was significantly superior in the IORT group: all control patients failed locally within 12 months, compared to >80% local control at 12 months in the IORT group (Sindelar and Kinsella 1986a).

The second study reported results obtained in patients with stage III or IV unresectable pancreatic cancer (some of whom thus had metastatic disease at the time of treatment), randomized to receive high dose external beam irradiation (60 Gy, split course) or 50 Gy external beam irradiation plus 25 Gy IORT boost. Both groups received intravenous 5-fluorouracil. The incidence of treatment-related complications was similar in the two groups. Median survival time in IORT and control patients was 8 months. Time to local disease progression was longer in the IORT group. For patients with local disease only (stage III) at the initiation of treatment, time to disease progression and survival were superior in the IORT group compared with the control group (Sindelar and Kinsella 1986b).

Unfortunately no new randomized trials are available in the literature. An interesting aspect that has been investigated is tumor response to

IORT and its radiologic patterns (Nishimura et al. 1987a,b). Recent reports emphasize the importance of including IORT as an adjuvant form of treatment following pancreatic tumor resection (Glaser et al. 1989; Heijmans et al. 1989; Hiraoka et al. 1989).

8.3 Treatment Protocol

A total of 35 patients treated with IORT during a 5-year period at the Clinica Universitaria de Navarra are analyzed below. The report concerns all patients seen with locally unresectable cancer of the pancreas and those with metastatic disease and associated severe abdominal pain. The locoregional treatment used consisted in any palliative surgical maneuver required, either biliary or biliary and gastrointestinal bypass, tumor biopsy, abdominal cavity disease staging, and tumor exposure for IORT. In general following omentectomy and mobilization of the stomach superiorly and the transverse colon inferiorly the tumor is exposed. The second and third portions of the duodenum are fixed structures that cannot be totally excluded from the IORT field if the tumor extends towards them. Those patients with proven localized disease were treated with fractionated external beam irradiation using four-field techniques and CT-planned dosimetric studies. Chemotherapy was occasionally given to patients with disseminated disease and some of those with a localized large tumor mass. The treatment regimen consisted of continuous infusion (for 4–5 days) of cisplatin and 5-fluorouracil.

8.4 Results

8.4.1 General Aspects of the Series

8.4.1.1 Patient Characteristics

For this study, patients were divided into two groups: those with localized disease and those with metastatic disease. The total number of patients treated was 35. Median age was 60 years, with a range of 21 to 81 years. There were 28 males and seven females. Karnofsky performance status was 70% or more in 16 patients (43%). The dominant initial symptom was abdominal pain (74%), followed by jaundice (51%) (Table 8.1).

Table 8.1. Patient characteristics

	Localized disease	Metastatic disease	Total (%)
No. of patients	25	10	35 (100)
Age			
Median	60	62	60
Range	21–81	45–75	21–81
Sex			
Male	20	8	28 (80)
Female	5	2	7 (20)
Karnofsky performance status			
>70%	12	4	16 (43)
<70%	13	6	19 (54)
Symptoms			
Abdominal pain	18	7	25 (74)
Jaundice	12	6	18 (51)
Weight loss	14	6	20 (57)
Others	13	3	16 (45)

8.4.1.2 Tumor Characteristics

Tumor diameter was 6 cm or more in nine cases (25%). The tumor was located in the head of the pancreas in 18 cases, the body in seven, and the tail in one. In nine cases the tumor location was classified as mixed due to the involvement of two of the above-mentioned pancreatic zones. Clinical and radiologic staging procedures showed 1 stage I tumor, 14 stage II, 10 stage III, and 10 stage IV. Nodal tumor involvement was confirmed surgically in seven patients with localized disease (Table 8.2).

8.4.1.3 Treatment Characteristics

Palliative surgical bypasses were performed in 27 cases: 16 combined biliary and gastrointestinal, five biliary alone, and six digestive alone. In the remaining eight cases surgery was performed to allow adequate tumor exposure for IORT. The IORT technique consisted in the use of a single field in 29 patients, while in six multiple adjacent fields were needed to cover the whole tumor volume. Cone diameter ranged from 5 to 10 cm. The electron energy selected was in most cases 18–20 MeV and the IORT single dose delivered was 15 Gy in 23 cases and 20 Gy in 18. The duodenum was partially included in the IORT field in seven cases.

External beam radiotherapy was given to all patients with localized disease and omitted in those with known metastases. The daily fractionation was 1.8–2 Gy 5 times per week, with the total

Table 8.2. Tumor characteristics

	Localized disease	Metastatic disease	Total (%)
Location			
Head	13	5	18 (51)
Body	6	1	7 (20)
Tail	–	1	1 (3)
Mixed	6	3	9 (25)
Size			
>6 cm	5	4	9 (25)
<6 cm	20	6	26 (75)
Stage			
I	1	–	1 (2)
II	14	–	14 (40)
III	10	–	10 (28)
IV	–	10	10 (28)
Nodes			
Positive	7	2	9 (25)
Negative	18	8	26 (75)

dose reaching 46 Gy (ten patients) or more (15 patients). Chemotherapy was used in 15 patients with localized and eight with metastatic disease (Table 8.3).

Table 8.3. Treatment characteristics

	Localized disease	Metastatic disease	Total (%)
Surgery			
Biliary and gastrointestinal bypass	9	7	16 (45)
Biliary bypass	4	1	5 (14)
Digestive bypass	6	0	6 (17)
Tumor exposure	6	2	8 (22)
IORT			
Fields[a]			
Single	23	6	29 (82)
Multiple	2	4	6 (18)
Cone diameter (cm)[a]			
5–6	8	9	17 (48)
7–8	15	2	17 (48)
9–10	4	3	7 (17)
Electron energy (MeV)[a]			
6–9	–	1	1 (2)
12–15	3	–	3 (7)
18–20	24	13	37 (91)
Total dose (Gy)[a]			
15	14	9	23 (56)
20	13	5	18 (44)
External beam radiotherapy			
46 Gy	15	–	15 (60)
50–55 Gy	10	–	10 (40)
Chemotherapy			
Yes	15	8	23 (65)
No	10	2	12 (35)

[a] A total of 41 IORT fields were treated

8.4.2 Toxicity and Complications

The clinical events related to the treatment program of surgery and IORT have been divided into acute and late complications. Early complications consisted of dumping syndrome ($n = 2$) peritonitis (1), gastrointestinal bleeding (4), postoperative fever (4), abdominal abscess (3), and a variety of minor problems (16). These episodes were all reversible with conservative treatment. Late complications seen after 4 or more months' follow-up included abdominal pain at the time of tumor progression (4), chronic diarrhea (3), gastrointestinal bleeding from duodenitis (2), biliary tract stenosis requiring surgical bypass (18 months after IORT) (1), cholangitis (1), and subocclusive intestinal crisis (2) (Table 8.4).

Table 8.4. Toxicity and complications

	Localized disease	Metastatic disease	Total
Acute complications			
Dumping syndrome	2	–	2
Peritonitis	1	–	1
GI bleeding	1	3	4
Abscess	2	1	3
Others	13	3	16
Late complications			
Abdominal pain	3	1	4
Diarrhea	2	1	3
GI bleeding	2	–	2
Biliary stenosis	1	–	1
Cholangitis	1	–	1
Subocclusion	2	–	2
Others	–	2	2

8.4.3 Patterns of Relapse

The patterns of relapse in unresected and/or metastatic pancreatic cancer have to be assessed in most instances by means of CT. In our series, patients were seen every 2–3 months and CT was performed on each occasion. In the group with metastatic disease at the time of treatment, survival was too short to evaluate local tumor control properly. Nevertheless, in this group of ten patients, one surviving 8 months had local tumor progression. In the group with locally unresectable disease, four had local tumor progression alone while three had local recurrence plus concomitant distant metastases. Distant failure as the first and

Table 8.5. Patterns of tumor progression

Disease at treatment	No. of patients	LP	LP + DM	DM
Localized	25	4	3	11
Metastatic	10	–	1	9
Total	35	4	4	20

Abbreviations: LP, local progression; DM, distant metastasis

only site of disease progression was seen in 11 patients (Table 8.5).

8.4.4 Survival

One patient in the group with metastatic disease is alive. The median survival time for this group is 4 months. In the group with locally unresectable disease, seven patients are alive (five are free of disease). The median survival time is 10 months (Fig. 8.1).

8.5 Conclusion

Our experience has been confined to the use of IORT in unresectable pancreatic cancer. The role of this treatment modality is well established and it is recognized worldwide that the pancreas is a site where IORT is feasible. Toxicities and complications are known, and there are marginal benefits in terms of survival as compared with external beam radiotherapy alone or in combination with systemic chemotherapy. A consistent positive finding is relief of abdominal pain, which was seen in 22 of 25 patients. This symptom was generally present at the time of diagnosis. As in other tumor sites, IORT seems to achieve more positive results in local control improvement and survival if tumor resection is performed: in fact the available data on adjuvant IORT in patients who have undergone tumor resection are rather encouraging. In general pancreatic cancer deserves further investigation in clinical oncology. There is an urgent need for an effective systemic treatment; such a treatment might be included in future programs in which external radiotherapy is given preoperatively in an effort to increase the resectability rate. IORT will be a valuable technique for those institutions with a particular interest in intensive locoregional cancer treatment.

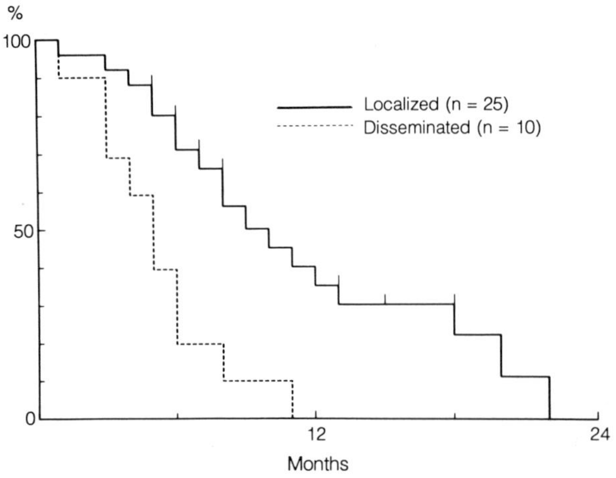

Fig. 8.1. Actuarial survival curves for patients with localized or disseminated unresectable pancreatic cancer, treated with IORT

References

Abe M, Takahashi M (1981) Intraoperative radiotherapy: the Japanese experience. Int J Radiat Oncol Biol Phys 7: 863–868

Abe M, Shibamoto Y, Takahasi M, Manabe T, Tobe T, Inamoto T (1987) Intraoperative radiotherapy in carcinoma of the stomach and pancreas. World J Surg 11: 459–464

Ahmadu-Suka F, Gillette EL, Withrow SJ, Husted PW, Nelson AW, Whiteman C (1988) Pathologic response of the pancreas and duodenum to experimental intraoperative radiation. Int J Radiat Oncol Biol Phys 14: 1197–1204

Bagne FR, Dobelbower RR, Milligan AJ, Bronn DG (1989) Treatment of cancer of the pancreas by intraoperative electron beam therapy: physical and biological aspects. Int J Radiat Oncol Biol Phys 16: 231–242

Bodner E, Glaser K (1989) First experiences with IORT in recurrent pancreatic cancer. Strahlenther Onkol 165: 775

Bodner E, Glaser K, Aufschnaiter M, Kohle W, Url M, Frommhold H (1986) Intraoperative radiation treatment of carcinoma of the pancreas. Initial clinical results. Dtsch Med Wochenschr 111: 892–896

Calvo FA, Santos M, Escude L, Hernandez JL, Chamorro A, Zornoza G, Voltas J (1987) Tratamiento del carcinoma avanzado de pancreas: experiencia inicial con radioterapia intraoperatoria. Oncologia 9: 121–128

Dobelbower RR, Abe M (1989) Intraoperative radiation therapy. CRC, Boca Raton, Fl

Dubois JB (1989) L'experience francaise dans la radiotherapie per-operatoire des cancers gastriques et pancreatiques. Ann Radiol 32: 487–488

Glaser K, Bocner E, Frommhold H (1989) Adjuvant IORT in resectable pancreatic cancer. Strahlenther Onkol 165: 774

Goldson AL, Ashaveri E, Espinoza MC et al. (1981) Single high dose intraoperative electrons for advanced stage pancreatic cancer: phase I pilot study. Int J Radiat Oncol Biol Phys 7: 869–874

Goldson AL, Ashayeri E, Collier-Manning J, King G, Nibhanupudy R (1989) Technical and clinical considerations for using the simultaneous delivery of intraoperative interstitial hyperthermia (IOHT) and intraoperative electrons (IORT) for pancreas cancer. Strahlenther Onkol 165: 774

Gunderson LL, Martin JK, Kvols LK et al. (1987) Intraoperative and external beam irradiation + 5-FU for locally advanced pancreatic cancer. Int J Radiat Oncol Biol Phys 13: 319–329

Hata K, Abe M, Nishimura A, Sakata S (1989) Intraoperative radiotherapy for carcinoma of the pancreas: analysis from Japan cross-institutional experience. Strahlenther Onkol 165: 772

Heijmans HJ, Hoeskstra HJ, Mehta DM (1989) Is adjuvant intra-operative radiotherapy (IORT) for resectable and unresectable pancreatic carcinoma worthwhile? Hepatogastroenterology 36: 474–477

Hiraoka T, Watanabe E, Mochinaga M, Tashiro S, Miyauchi Y, Nakamura I, Yokoyama I (1984) Intraoperative irradiation combined with radical resection for cancer of the head of the pancreas. World J Surg 8: 766–771

Hiraoka T, Nakamura I, Tashiro S, Miyauchi Y (1989) Intraoperative radiation therapy for pancreatic cancer in Japan. In: Dobelbower RR, Abe M (eds) Intraoperative radiation therapy. CRC, Boca Raton, Fl, pp 181–194

Hoekstra HJ, Restrepo C, Kinsella TJ, Sindelar WF (1988) Histopathological effects of intraoperative radiotherapy on pancreas and adjacent tissues: a postmortem analysis. J Surg Oncol 37: 104–108

Hoekstra HJ, Mehta DM, Heijmans HJ (1989) The role of intraoperative electron beam radiotherapy (IORT) in the treatment of unresectable pancreatic cancer. Strahlenther Onkol 165: 774

Hoopes PJ, Gillette EL, Withrow WJ (1987) Intraoperative irradiation of the canine abdominal aorta and vena cava. Int J Radiat Oncol Biol Phys 13: 715–722

Huguier M, Schlienger M, Houry S, Lacaine F, Charron R (1987) La radiotherapie peroperatoire dans les cancers du pancreas. Presse Med 16: 2009–2012

Kamata R, Maeno T, Sanuki E, Kumagai Y, Saito T, Takashima H (1989) Experience with IOR for advanced pancreatic carcinoma. Strahlenther Onkol 165: 773

Kiel KD, Kramer T, Rosenman D (1989) Intraoperative radiation therapy for carcinoma of the pancreas: the early experience at Rush Presbyterian St. Luke's Medical Center. Strahlenther Onkol 165: 776

Kita M, Okawa T, Tanaka M, Ikeda M, Hanyu F (1989) Multimodal treatment for pancreatic cancer. The efficacy of intraoperative radiotherapy. Strahlenther Onkol 165: 772

Matsuda T, Tanaka Y (1989) Intraoperative radiation therapy in combination with computer-controlled conformation radiotherapy for pancreatic cancer. In: Dobelbower RR, Abe M (eds) Intraoperative radiation therapy. CRC, Boca Raton, Fl, pp 195–216

Merrik HW, Milligan AJ, Greenblatt SH, Dobelbower RR (1989) Clinical experience with intraoperative interstitial hyperthermia in conjunction with intraoperative radiation therapy for deep seated tumors. Strahlenther Onkol 165: 774

Nakano M, Nishimura A, Iida K, Oohara K, Todoroki T, Iwasaki Y (1989) Intraoperative radiotherapy for pancreatic cancer. 15-years' experience and its clinical significance. Strahlenther Onkol 165: 772

Nishimura A, Nakano M, Otsu H et al. (1984) Intraoperative radiotherapy for advanced carcinoma of the pancreas. Cancer 54: 2375–2384

Nishimura A, Otsu H, Itoh I, Sakata S, Iwabuchi K, Kurata N, Nakano M (1987a) Response of pancreatic tumor to intraoperative radiotherapy: medical imaging and pathologic system approach. J Comput Tomogr 11: 5–15

Nishimura A, Otsu H, Itoh I, Sakata S, Iida K, Nakano M, Furuse T (1987b) Prognostic significance of pancreatic tumor regression after intraoperative radiotherapy. Strahlenther Onkol 163: 350–356

Roldan GE, Gunderson LL, Nagorney DM et al. (1988) External beam versus intraoperative and external beam irradiation for locally advanced pancreatic cancer. Cancer 61: 1110–1116

Shipley WU, Wood WC, Tepper JE et al. (1984) Intraoperative electron beam irradiation for patients with unresectable pancreatic carcinoma. Ann Surg 200: 289–296

Sindelar WF, Kinsella TJ (1986a) Randomized trial of intraoperative radiotherapy in resected carcinoma of the pancreas. Int J Radiat Oncol Biol Phys 12 [Suppl 1]: 148

Sindelar WF, Kinsella TJ (1986b) Randomized trial of intraoperative raidotherapy in unresectable carcinoma of the pancreas. Int J Radiat Oncol Biol Phys 12 [Suppl 1]: 148

Sindelar WF, Tepper JE, Travis EL (1982a) Tolerance of bile duct to intraoperative irradiation. Surgery 92: 533–540

Sindelar WF, Tepper JE, Travis EL, Terrill R (1982b) Tolerance of retroperitoneal structures to intraoperative radiation. Ann Surg 196: 601–608

Sindelar WF, Morrow B, Travis EL, Tepper J, Merkel AB, Kranda K, Terrill R (1983) Effects of intraoperative electron irradiation in the dog on cell turnover in intact and surgically-anastomosed aorta and intestine. Int J Radiat Oncol Biol Phys 9: 523–532

Sindelar WF, Kinsella TJ, Mayer RJ (1985a) Cancer of the pancreas. In: De Vita VT, Hellman S, Rosemberg SA (eds) Principles and practice of oncology, 2nd edn. JB Lippincott, Philadelphia, pp 722–726

Sindelar WF, Kinsella TJ, Hoekstra HJ, Tochner ZA, Smith R, Maher MM (1985b) Duodenal hemorrhage as a complication of intraoperative radiotherapy for unresectable carcinomas of the pancreas. Proc Am Soc Clin Oncol 4: 277

Sindelar WF, Hoekstra HJ, Restrepo C, Kinsella TJ (1986) Pathologic tissue changes following intraoperative radiotherapy. Am J Clin Oncol 9: 504–509

Tanaka Y, Matsuda T, Takeshita N, Okamoto A, Tabata I (1989) Intraoperative radiotherapy of pancreatic carcinoma: results of combined modality with postoperative conformation radiotherapy. Strahlenther Onkol 165: 773

Tepper JE, Sindelar WF, Travis EL, Terrill R, Padikas T (1983) Tolerance of canine anastomosis to intraoperative radiation therapy. Int J Radiat Oncol Biol Phys 9: 987–992

Tepper JE, Shipley WU, Warshaw AL, Nardi GL, Wood WC, Orlow EL (1987) The role of misonidazole combined with intraoperative radiation therapy in the treatment of pancreatic carcinoma. J Clin Oncol 5: 579–584

Willett CG, Shipley WU, Warshaw AL, Tepper JE, Wood WC, Nardi GL, Stracher MA (1989) Intraoperative radiation therapy for locally advanced pancreatic cancer. Strahlenther Onkol 165: 773

Willich N, Teichmann R, Krimmel K, Naujokat B, Denecke H, Wend T, Rohloff R (1988) Intraoperative electron irradiation of malignant pancreatic tumors. Initial experiences at Grobhadern. Strahlenther Onkol 164: 187–194

Willich N, Deneke H, Krimmel K, Grab J (1989a) The Munich experience in intraoperative irradiation therapy of pancreatic cancer. Ann Radiol 324: 484–486

Willich N, Denecke H, Naujokat B, Krimmel K (1989b) First experience at Grobhadern in IORT of malignant pancreatic tumors. Strahlenther Onkol 165: 776

Wood WC, Shipley WU, Gunderson LL, Cohen AM, Nardi GL (1982) Intraoperative irradiation for unresectable pancreatic carcinoma. Cancer 49: 1272–1275.

Yasue M (1988) Intraoperative radiation therapy of adenocarcinoma of the pancreas. Gan To Kagaku Ryoho 15: 770–776

9 Colorectal Cancer

Felipe A. Calvo, Ignacio Azinovic, Fernando Pardo, José L. Hernández, and Javier Alvarez-Cienfuegos

CONTENTS

9.1 Introduction 65
9.2 Previous Experiences 65
9.2.1 Tissue Tolerance Studies 65
9.2.2 Clinical Results 66
9.3 Treatment Protocol 67
9.4 Results 68
9.4.1 Patient, Tumor, and Treatment Characteristics 68
9.4.2 Toxicity and Complications 68
9.4.3 Patterns of Tumor Recurrence 70
9.4.4 Outcome and Survival Data 71
9.5 Conclusion 71
References 71

9.1 Introduction

It is accepted that the incorporation of external beam radiotherapy in the management of rectal cancer promotes pelvic disease control (Gunderson 1987). The results of preoperative and postoperative radiotherapy trials, with or without chemotherapy, are consistent with high local tumor control rates (Dosoretz et al. 1983; Gunderson and Martenson 1988). Phase III trials have established the value of combined modality treatment in rectal cancer (Gastrointestinal Tumor Study Group 1986). In cancer of the colon the role of external beam radiotherapy remains controversial, in part due to the difficulty in delivering high doses of radiation in abdominal areas (Gunderson and Martenson 1989). On the other hand, cancer of the colon is a recently established indication for adjuvant chemoimmunotherapy (Moertel et al. 1990).

Felipe A. Calvo, Dr., Director and Consultant, Ignacio Azinovic, Dr., Radiotherapy Division, Department of Oncology, Fernando Pardo, Dr., Consultant, José L. Hernández, Dr., Consultant, Javier Alvarez-Cienfuegos, Dr., Consultant, Department of Surgery, Clinica Universitaria de Navarra, 31080 Pamplona, Spain

Use of IORT for colorectal cancer has shed new light on the treatment modality, in terms of both concepts and technique (Gunderson et al. 1983a). For example, a correlation has been established between local control and excellence of surgery (Tepper et al. 1984b), survival following primary and recurrent disease has been analyzed (Gunderson et al. 1988), and it has been ascertained that the incidence of postoperative complications is not increased in IORT patients (Tepper et al. 1984); finally, quality control parameters have been established in IORT studies (Tepper et al. 1986a). IORT was initially considered for the treatment only of unresectable or known residual disease (Gunderson et al. 1983b). Such indications will include a significant number of patients with recurrent disease and a poor long-term prognosis. In fact, however, by reference to colorectal cancer it is possible to demonstrate that IORT should be integrated into the management of early and intermediate tumor stages rather than being limited to the rescue of recurrences or locally advanced tumors. Colorectal cancer is indeed a reasonable model for testing locoregional intensification programs in a multidisciplinary treatment approach (Gunderson et al. 1983c).

9.2 Previous Experiences

9.2.1 Tissue Tolerance Studies

Animal studies have analyzed the tolerance of pelvic organs and structures to experimental IORT alone or in combination with fractionated external beam irradiation.

During colorectal cancer surgery the target areas selected for IORT will in most instances include large vessels (iliac artery and vein), pelvic side walls, and the sciatic nerve. Occasionally the ureter or a portion of the bladder or prostate is involved by or in close contact with tumor, and therefore will be included in the IORT field. In the case of recurrent tumors the presacral space is the area most frequently involved by tumor. Vessels and/or ureters might also be near to or involved by tumor. Tissue tolerance has been analyzed for the ureter (Gillette et al. 1989), peripheral nerves (Le Coteur et al. 1989), bone (Powers et al. 1989), and large vessels (Hoopes et al. 1987). When single doses of IORT alone are used, the bladder and peripheral nerves appear to tolerate up to 20 Gy without significant toxicity (Hoekstra et al. 1984). However, it has been shown that when IORT boost and external beam irradiation are used in combination, the IORT component of the irradiation treatment has to be decreased to 10–15 Gy. Clinical practice has confirmed that moderate doses of IORT in combination with external beam irradiation are acceptably tolerated by normal tissues in the pelvis and that local control rates are high enough to render unnecessary an increase in the dose of any of the components of radiotherapy programs.

An important collection of data analyzed with regard to toxicity has been reported by the Mayo Clinic Group (SHAW et al. 1987). The study reviewed the experience over a 5-year period (1981–1985) using IORT in patients with pelvic tumors. The vast majority had colorectal cancer (38 out of 51). The treatment program combined surgery, IORT (10–25 Gy; median dose 17.5 Gy), and preoperative or postoperative external pelvic irradiation (median dose 50.4 Gy). Twenty-nine (57%) patients developed toxicity, and in 18 cases (35% of all cases) IORT was an etiologic factor. One patient died from an arterial fistula with massive gastrointestinal bleeding, possibly related to IORT. Peripheral lower extremity neuropathy was seen in 16 patients (32%), but this finding was present in almost half of the patients treated to the pelvic side wall. The clinical picture was characterized by unilateral pain (100%), numbness (69%), and/or weakness (90%). Resolution of symptoms occurred in 38% of patients with pain, but in only 13% of those with weakness. Ureteral obstruction was the second most common IORT toxicity. Twenty-three ureters in 19 patients received IORT (16 unobstructed by tumor, seven obstructed). Subsequently, 10 of the 16 patients with initially unobstructed ureters (63%) developed hydronephrosis, whereas three with initially obstructed ureters had resolution of their tumor-associated hydronephrosis. The remaining toxicities were attributed primarily to external beam irradiation with or without surgery; they included pelvic abscess, small bowel obstruction, and delayed wound healing.

9.2.2 Clinical Results

The initial report from the Massachusetts General Hospital group emphasized the importance of the assessment of complications resulting from the use of new treatment modalities (Tepper et al. 1984a). The study compared severe complications occurring after IORT in patients with locally advanced rectal cancer (primary or recurrent disease) with those in two similar groups of patients treated with surgery alone or preoperative radiotherapy plus surgery. The authors found complication rates to be higher in all irradiated patients than in those who had undergone surgery alone (results not statistically significant). When the pelvic complications involving soft tissues were analyzed, the patients with local recurrences treated with a combination of surgery, external beam radiotherapy, and IORT were found to have the highest complication rate (41%). The study showed increased complication rates in patients with locally advanced rectal cancer and with the complexity of the treatment itself. No increase in sepsis or infections was found.

The two centers in the United States with the greatest experience in the use of IORT for the treatment of colorectal cancer have updated their results several times (Gunderson et al. 1983a, 1988; Tepper et al. 1986b). At the Massachusetts General Hospital a total of 58 patients were treated with IORT; 36 had primary locally advanced disease and 22 had recurrent disease (Tepper et al. 1989). All patients in this series received preoperative external beam irradiation and after a rest period (approximately 4 weeks) were operated upon. One local failure was observed in 20 patients with primary locally advanced tumors that were completely resected, while two such failures occurred in 16 patients in the same category with partial tumor resection. As regards local failures in patients with recurrent tumors, two occurred in nine cases of complete resection, six in eight cases of partial resection, and four in five cases without resection. The 3-year actuarial survival rate is 58% in the primary disease group and 32% in the recurrent disease group. Tepper et al. concluded that the local control and survival results in the primary tumors appeared favorable compared with the other series reported in the literature and suggested some benefit from the use of IORT. For patients treated for local recurrences, local control and long-term survival could be obtained, but the results were not as encouraging as for the primary tumors. The complication rate in this report was low, particularly with regard to ureteral and nerve damage.

The Mayo Clinic experience over a 5-year period has recently been reported (GUNDERSON et al. 1988). The treatment program included combination of external pelvic irradiation and IORT boost (10–20 Gy), with or without 5-fluorouracil. There were 36 cases of recurrent disease and 15 of primary disease. At the time of the report 30 of the 51 patients were alive and 22 were free of disease. Among 44 patients at risk for more than 1 year, local progression has occurred within the IORT field in one and within the external beam field in eight. All local failures have been detected in patients with recurrences or with gross residual disease after partial resection, and the risk was lower in patients who received 5-fluorouracil during external beam irradiation (1 of 11, 9%, vs 6 of 31, 19%). The incidence of distant metastasis is high in patients with recurrence. Analyzing the toxicity and complications, an important finding was neuropathy in patients treated with IORT for pelvic tumors. In this report 37 such patients had a follow-up of more than 1 year and were at risk for the development of neuropathy. The clinical characteristics of neuropathy were pain in 12 cases (severe in three), sensory deficits in eight (no severe cases seen), and motor deficits in seven (one severe case). The symptoms resolved in five out of 12 patients with pain and one out of seven patients with motor deficits. The authors concluded that expansion and refinement of IORT approaches are warranted, but randomized trials will be the ultimate test of whether observed differences in local control and survival are true advantages obtained from the integration of IORT in treatment management, or merely due to a difference in case selection.

A more selective analysis of toxicity data has been reported recently (SHAW et al. 1990)

9.3 Treatment Protocol

This chapter reviews the clinical experience obtained with IORT during a 6-year period in patients with locally advanced colorectal cancer. All Patients who had local disease underwent surgical tumor exposure and/or resection and received an IORT dose of more than 10 Gy. Pretreatment studies included: history and physical examination, routine blood tests, liver enzymes, CEA levels, chest x-ray, barium enema, abdominopelvic CT scan, and rectosigmoidoscopy plus biopsy. Bone scan and liver sonography were optional.

For the purpose of analysis, cases have been grouped into three categories: group P, comprising primary colorectal fixed or advanced tumors treated by surgical resection, IORT boost to the tumor bed, and pre- or postoperative external beam irradiation; group R, comprising localized recurrences following surgery in patients without previous external beam radiotherapy in the area of recurrence; group RR, comprising localized recurrences in previously irradiated zones.

The surgical procedure performed was the most radical one possible in each individual case. Surgery for tumor exposure alone or minor resection was avoided, except in those cases in which a radical surgical alternative did not exist.

External beam radiotherapy consisted in all cases in large pelvic field irradiation, including the perineum in all recurrent cases and in most primary tumors with low rectal locations. The radiation beam employed was 15 MV photons, with an AP-PA technique in most preoperative cases and a three- or four-field technique in postoperative cases. Daily fractionation was conventional (1.8–2 Gy/day). Total doses ranged from 40 to 50 Gy. In general, 40 Gy was reserved for patients receiving simultaneous chemotherapy preoperatively. Primary tumors involving the sigmoid zone received large field irradiation that included the primary site, the pelvis, and para-aortic areas.

More recently chemotherapy was administered to patients with initially advanced primary tumors or local recurrences, simultaneously with pelvic irradiation. The program consisted in carboplatin 50 mg/m^2 i.v. and 5-fluorouracil 1500 mg i.v. given by continuous 24-h infusion over 3–4 days at the initiation of irradiation and at the end of it.

The IORT technique was similar to that employed in the other tumor sites. In general, the use of one single field to encompass the tumor mass or tumor bed area was encouraged. The energy employed had to include within the 90% isodose curve margins of normal tissue equal to the thickness of tumor left after surgery. The total IORT dose was in the range of 10–15 Gy for patients not previously irradiated, and 15–20 Gy in those in whom disease was recurrent (Fig. 9.1).

Following the completion of the treatment program, patients were followed up every 3 months with a clinical consultation, physical examination, blood tests, abdominopelvic CT scan, and any other optional study deemed necessary. Presacral masses detected by CT in the follow-up period were investigated by aspiration cytology if an increase in size (compared with the postsurgical baseline scan) was detected and/or there was associated pelvic pain. In the presence of unexplained pelvic pain, electrophysiologic nerve conduction studies were done.

9.4 Results

9.4.1 Patient, Tumor, and Treatment Characteristics

The total number of patients analyzed in this report is 49. Age ranged from 37 to 80 years, with a median of 56 years. Twenty-eight of the patients were males and 21, females. Karnofsky performance status was greater than 70% in 41 patients. Common symptoms at the time of diagnosis were pain and bleeding. Elevated CEA values were also observed. Patient characteristics are shown in Table 9.1.

Adenocarcinoma was the tumor histology reported in 47 cases. In all but two of the cases in which the degree of differentiation was established, tumors were found to be well or moderately differentiated. The primary tumor site was the rectosigmoid area in 42 cases, the ascending colon in five, and the descending colon in two. The maximum diameter of the primary tumor or the recurrent mass was greater than 4 cm in 38 cases (Table 9.2).

The surgical approach was quite conventional in patients with primary tumors, including low anterior and abdominoperineal resections in most cases; exenterations were mostly performed in recurrent cases. External beam radiotherapy was given preoperatively to 23 patients. The total dose was more than 40 Gy in all cases. Simultaneous chemotherapy with radiation therapy was given in eight cases (Table 9.3).

The technical aspects of IORT included the use of a single field in 46 cases, with a wide range of cone sizes from 5 to 10 cm. In 42 fields, the energy

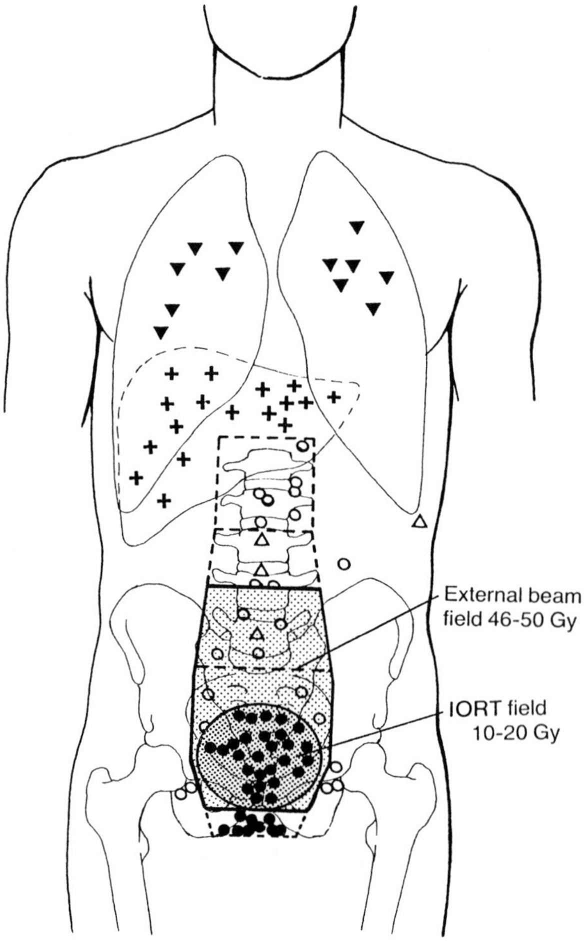

Fig. 9.1. Diagram showing the integration of IORT boost and external beam irradiation

employed ranged from 6 to 12 MeV. Normal pelvic tissues and structures in some instances included in the IORT field due to either tumor involvement or technical difficulties were the ureter, bladder, prostate, rectum, duodenum (in a mesenteric root nodal recurrence), and sigmoid colon (Table 9.4).

9.4.2 Toxicity and Complications

A detailed analysis of all toxicities and clinical problems related to the treatment program has been performed. A variety of observations were noted, including infectious processes and perineal fistulas that might be related to the overall treatment approach. External beam irradiation might be the principal cause of long-term findings such as ileitis, cystitis, and subocclusive intestinal

Table 9.1. Patient characteristics

	Primary disease	Recurrent disease	Reirradiation	Total
Number	21	21	7	49
Age (years)				
Mean	61	54	52	56
Range	37–77	37–80	36–65	37–80
Sex				
Male	9	14	5	28
Female	12	7	2	21
Karnofsky performance status				
>70%	18	18	5	41
<70%	3	3	2	8
Symptoms				
Pain	9	12	6	27
Bleeding	14	4	6	24
Elevated CEA	4	9	4	17

Table 9.2. Tumor characteristics

	P	R	RR	Total
Histology				
Adenocarcinoma	20	20	7	47
Carcinoma	1	1	–	2
Differentiation				
Well differentiated	4	4	1	9
Moderately differentiated	12	11	5	28
Poorly differentiated	1	1	–	2
Unknown	4	5	1	10
Location				
Ascending colon	3	2	–	5
Descending colon	–	2	–	2
Rectosigmoid	18	17	7	42
Size				
≥4 cm	16	15	7	38
≤4 cm	5	6	–	11

Abbreviations: P, primary disease; R, recurrent disease; RR, radiation recurrence

Table 9.3. Treatment characteristics

	P	R	RR	Total
Surgery				
Low anterior resection	10	10	1	21
Abdominoperineal resection	9	2	–	11
Tumor exposure	1	4	–	5
Pelvic exenteration	1	3	5	9
Transperineal resection	–	2	1	3
Residual disease				
Microscopic	19	17	–	36
Macroscopic	2	4	7	13
Radiotherapy				
Preoperative	14	9	–	23
Postoperative	7	12	–	19
Total dose				
40–45 Gy	9	11	–	20
46–50 Gy	12	10	–	22
Chemotherapy				
Simultaneous	4	4	–	8
Not given	16	13	4	33
Preoperative	–	3	2	5

Abbreviations: P, primary disease; R, recurrent disease; RR, radiation recurrence

Table 9.4. Technical details of IORT

	P	R	RR	Total
Number of fields				
Single	21	19	6	46
Multiple	–	2	1	3
Cone diameter (cm)				
5	–	3	2	5
6	7	7	–	14
7	8	1	2	11
8	3	7	3	13
9	2	3	–	5
10	1	2	1	4
Electron energy (MeV)				
6	4	1	–	5
9	13	3	3	17
12	3	12	5	20
15	–	2	1	3
20	1	6	–	7
Total dose (Gy)				
<15	8	1	–	9
15	11	22	6	39
20	2	–	2	4
Tissues included				
Ureter	1	4	–	5
Bladder	3	4	–	7
Prostate	1	–	–	1
Rectum	–	3	–	3
Duodenum	–	1	–	1
Sigmoid colon	–	1	–	1

Abbreviations: P, primary disease; R, recurrent disease; RR, radiation recurrence

crisis. The combination of IORT and external beam radiotherapy, with or without surgical tissue manipulation, might be the single most important factor responsible for the development of ureteral stenosis, pelvic pain due to neuropathy, and delayed wound healing. As shown in Table 9.5, there was a much higher rate of complications in patients with recurrences than in those with primary tumors. An important finding in our series was massive perineal bleeding, observed at late follow-up (8 and 12 months) in two patients with apparently stable disease.

9.4.3 Patterns of Tumor Recurrence

The median follow-up time for the entire series is 13 months, with a range from 1+ to 58+ months.

Table 9.5. Toxicity and complications observed

	P	R	RR	Total
Abscess	–	3	1	4
Subocclusive crisis	2	3	1	6
Postoperative fever	4	3	2	9
Perineal fistula	1	6	3	10
Pelvic pain	–	6	2	8
Ureteral stenosis	3	3	–	6
Duodenitis	–	1	–	1
Radiation ileitis	2	1	–	3
Radiation cystitis	–	1	–	1
Delayed wound healing	–	2	–	2
Neuropathy	–	1	3	4
Long-term perineal bleeding	–	2	–	2

Abbreviations: P, primary disease; R, recurrent disease; RR, radiation recurrence

Table 9.6. Patterns of tumor recurrences

	P	R	RR	Total
Local failure alone	–	2[a]	2[c]	4
Local failure + distant metastasis	–	4[b]	2[d]	6
Distant metastasis alone	4	4	1	9

Abbreviations: P, primary disease; R, recurrent disease; RR, radiation recurrence
[a] One patient with macroscopic residual disease
[b] Three patients with macroscopic residual disease
[c] Both patients with macroscopic residual disease
[d] One patient with macroscopic residual disease

At the time of this analysis a total of 19 patients have had documented tumor progression – ten local failures and 15 distant dissemination (six have been mixed failures) (Table 9.6). Local failures have been seen only in patients with recurrent disease, and seven out of ten had macroscopic residual disease at the time of surgery. The first site for distant disease progression has been the liver in nine cases, lymph nodes in two, bone in one, and anastomotic stump in two.

9.4.4 Outcome and Survival Data

A total of 19 patients have died during the follow-up period. All patients with recurrent disease in a previously irradiated zone died within 18 months after IORT, with a median survival time of 5 months. Of the 21 patients with recurrent disease treated with the complete program, 11 died and the actuarial survival rate is 20% projected at 6 years. In the locally advanced primary tumor group, one patient died of progressive disease, but three patients are alive with disease at 5, 7, and 12 months' follow up (Fig. 9.2).

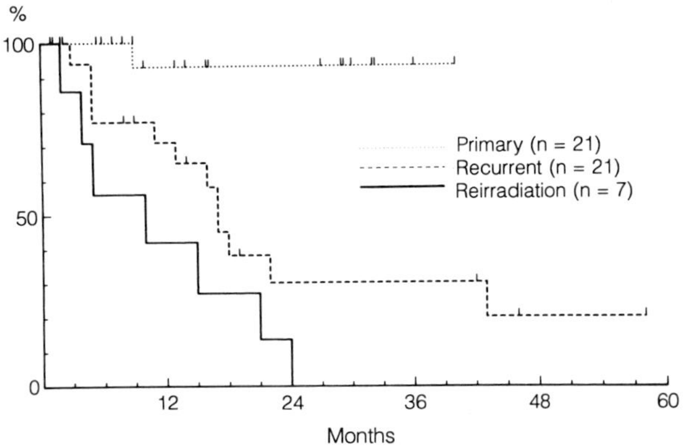

Fig. 9.2. Actuarial survival curves for the groups of colorectal cancer patients treated with IORT

9.5 Conclusion

Investigations in several institutions around the world have proven the integration of IORT in the treatment of locally advanced colorectal cancer to be feasible and well tolerated. Comparable local control rates have been obtained by those groups using similar treatment programs, and seem to be higher than the local control rates expected without electron boost. Colorectal cancer is a disease model for testing the possible value of locoregional as well as intensified systemic treatment programs. The initial suggestions that tumor control in IORT trials might be related to disease status (better results in primary than in recurrent tumors), amount of residual disease left after surgery, and primary tumor stage have been confirmed whenever such analysis has been performed. There are occasional technical limitations on the use of IORT for pelvic tumors, but the technique would be satisfactory in more than 80% of patients considered for treatment. Phase III trials have now been activated in a multi-institutional context. It will be an exceptional situation in modern clinical oncology for a boosting radiotherapy technique to be tested in a randomized study.

References

Dosoretz DE, Gunderson LL, Hoskins B et al. (1983) Preoperative irradiation for localized carcinoma of the rectum and rectosigmoid: patterns of failure, survival, and future treatment strategies. Cancer 52: 814–818
Gastrointestinal Tumor Study Group (1986) Survival after postoperative combination treatment of colorectal cancer. N Engl J Med 315: 1294–1295
Gillette SL, Gillette EL, Powers BE et al. (1989) Ureteral injury following experimental intraoperative irradiation. Int J Radiat Oncol Biol Phys 17: 791–798
Gunderson LL (1987) Colorectal cancer. In: Perez CA, Brady LW (eds) Principles and practice of radiation oncology. JB Lippincott, Philadelphia, pp 813–829

Gunderson LL, Martenson JA (1988) Irradiation of adenocarcinoma of the gastrointestinal tract. Front Radiat Ther Oncol 22: 127–148

Gunderson LL, Martenson JA (1989) Gastrointestinal tract radiation tolerance. Front Radiat Ther Oncol 23: 277–298

Gunderson LL, Cohen AM, Dosoretz DE et al. (1983a) Residual, unresectable, or recurrent colorectal cancer: external beam irradiation and intraoperative electron beam boost +/− resection. Int J Radiat Oncol Biol Phys 9: 1597–1606

Gunderson LL, Tepper JE, Bigg PJ et al. (1983b) Intraoperative +/− external beam irradiation. Curr Probl Cancer 7: 1–69

Gunderson LL, Tepper JE, Dosoretz DE et al. (1983c) Patterns of failure after treatment of gastrointestinal cancer. Cancer Treat Symp 2: 181–197

Gunderson LL, Martin JK, Beart RW et al. (1988) External beam and intraoperative electron irradiation for locally advanced colorectal cancer. Ann Surg 27: 52–60

Hoekstra HJ, Kisella TJ, Maher M et al. (1985) Treatment complications related to intraoperative radiotherapy. Proc Am Soc Clin Oncol 4: 254

Hoopes PJ, Gillette EL, Withrow SJ (1987) Intraoperative irradiation of the canine abdominal aorta and vena cava. Int J Radiat Oncol Biol Phys 13: 715–722

Kinsella TJ, Sidellar WF, De Luca AM, Terrill R (1985) Tolerance of peripheral nerve to intraoperative radiotherapy (IORT): clinical and experimental studies. Int J Radiat Oncol Biol Phys 11: 1579–1585

Kinsella TJ, Sidellar WF, De Luca AM et al. (1988) Tolerance of the canine bladder to intraoperative radiation therapy: an experimental study. Int J Radiat Oncol Phys 14: 939–946

Le Coteur RA, Gillette EL, Powers BE et al. (1989) Peripheral neuropathies following experimental intraoperative radiation therapy (IORT). Int J Radiat Oncol Biol Phys 17: 583–590

Moertel CG, Fleming TR, McDonald JS et al. (1990) Levamisole and fluorourcil for adjuvant therapy of resected colon carcinoma. N Engl J Med 322: 352–358

Powers BE, Gillette EL, McHesney SL et al. (1989) Bone necrosis and tumor induction following experimental intraoperative irradiation. Int J Radiat Biol Phys 17: 559–567

Shaw EG, Gunderson LL, Martin JK et al. (1987) Toxicity and results of intraoperative radiation therapy for primary unresectable and recurrent pelvic malignancies. Am J Clin Oncol 10: 105

Shaw EG, Gunderson LL, Martin JK et al. (1990) Peripheral nerve and ureteral tolerance of intraoperative radiation therapy: clinical and dose response analysis. Radiother Oncol 18: 247–255

Sindelar WF, Morrow BM, Travis EL et al. (1983) Effects of intraoperative electron irradiation in the dog on cell turnover in intact and surgically-anastomosed aorta and intestine. Int J Radiat Oncol Biol Phys 9: 523–532

Tepper JE, Gunderson LL, Orlow E et al. (1984a) Complications of intraoperative radiation therapy. Int J Radiat Oncol Biol Phys 10: 1831–1839

Tepper JE, Wood WC, Cohen WC et al. (1984b) Intraoperative radiation therapy. In: De Vita VT, Hellman S, Rosenberg S (eds). Important advances in oncology. JB Lippincott, Philadelphia, pp 226–242

Tepper JE, Gunderson LL, Goleson AL et al. (1986a) Quality control parameters of intraoperative radiation therapy. Int Radiat Oncol Biol Phys 12: 1687–1695

Tepper JE, Cohem AM, Wood WC et al. (1986b) Intraoperative electron beam radiotherapy in the treatment of unresectable rectal cancer. Arch Surg 121: 421–423

Tepper JE, Wood WC, Cohem AM (1989) Treatment of locally advanced rectal cancer with external beam radiation, surgical resection, and intraoperative radiation therapy. Int J Radiat Oncol Biol Phys 16: 1437–1444

10 Bladder Cancer

Felipe A. Calvo, Oscar Abuchaibe, Javier Aristu, Javier Zudiare, and José María Berián

CONTENTS

10.1	Introduction	73
10.2	Previous Experiences	73
10.2.1	Tissue Tolerance Studies	73
10.2.2	Clinical Results	74
10.3	Treatment Protocol	74
10.4	Results	76
10.4.1	Patient, Tumor, and Treatment Characteristics	76
10.4.2	Pathologic Findings After Cystectomy	76
10.4.3	Patterns of Tumor Recurrence and Survival Data	76
10.5	Conclusion	77
	References	77

10.1 Introduction

The management of invasive bladder cancer has altered over the last decade (Richie et al. 1989). Neoadjuvant chemotherapy has attracted increasing interest, while the role of radiation therapy is still controversial (Raghavan 1988; Quilty and Duncan 1986). Radical surgery achieves local disease control in some patients, and these local control rates have been improved upon in studies in which combined treatment was explored, generally using preoperative radiotherapy (Skinner and Lieskovsky 1984; Montie et al. 1984; Parsons and Million 1988; Bloom et al. 1982). Chemotherapy might prevent systemic disease development at the same time as surgical resection rates are being improved (Sternberg et al. 1988). In this era of systemic and local treatment intensification, the issue of organ preservation in bladder cancer patients has been repeatedly raised (Eapen et al. 1989). Radiotherapy has been proven to produce a modest rate of long-term survival in patients with invasive bladder cancer, in many cases referred for irradiation due to poor general status or other conditions that contraindicated radical surgery (Shipley et al. 1985). Moreover, some excellent results in terms of organ preservation have been achieved using sophisticated radiotherapy techniques such as brachytherapy alone or in combination with external beam radiotherapy (Van der Werf-Messing et al. 1983).

The modern approach to organ preservation trials including radiotherapy is based upon strict selection criteria: only those patients who exhibit a complete tumor response after initial induction therapy are candidates for high dose external beam radiotherapy in an effort to preserve the bladder (Marks et al. 1988). Within this frame work, IORT is an attractive boosting modality. IORT can accurately treat tumors located in the lateral and posterior bladder walls, and avoid irradiation to the small bowel and rectum (Shipley et al. 1987).

In our institution we have explored the integration of IORT in a multidisciplinary treatment program for locally advanced bladder cancer using preoperative radiotherapy and more recently a combination of neoadjuvant chemotherapy and preoperative irradiation. An important aspect of our experience has been the possibility it has afforded to analyze the cystectomy specimen and to correlate the pathologic findings with the previous treatment program. This information is of particular value for the development of clinical trials using IORT as a boosting modality in organ preservation protocols (Calvo et al. 1990).

10.2 Previous Experiences

10.2.1 Tissue Tolerance Studies

At the National Cancer Institute (Kinsella et al. 1988) an experimental study of bladder cancer

Felipe A. Calvo, Dr., Director and Consultant, Oscar Abuchaibe, Dr., Javier Aristu, Dr., Radiotherapy Division, Department of Oncology, Javier Zudaire, Dr., Consultant, José M. Berián, Dr., Consultant, Department of Urology, Clinica Universitaria de Navarra, 31080 Pamplona, Spain tolerance to IORT employed a large animal model to assess acute and late radiation effects. After cystectomy IORT was delivered using a 5-cm circular cone and a 12 MeV electron beam to an area including the trigone, ureteral orifices, and proximal urethra, with escalating single doses of 0, 20, 25, 30, 35, and 40 Gy. No fractionated external beam radiotherapy was delivered. Dogs were electively sacrificed at 1 and 2 years, or followed clinically for a minimum of 4 years. Obstruction of a ureteral orifice and renal failure secondary to bilateral hydronephrosis was seen in 3 out of 15 dogs that received 25, 35, and 40 Gy. Serial cystometry demonstrated no major loss of bladder contractility or volume. At autopsy, histologic changes comprising mucosa thinning and telangiectasia with submucosal fibrosis were confined to the IORT field and appeared to be dose related. The bladder epithelium remained intact at all doses. The ureterovesical junction in animals receiving 20 Gy showed mild fibrosis of the lamina propria and moderate chronic inflammation. Above 20 Gy the histologic changes at the ureterovesical junction were pronounced, with gross stenosis in three animals. The authors concluded that the bladder trigone will tolerate 20 Gy IORT without major clinical sequelae. In a recent report (Hoekstra et al. 1989) an interesting and new observation has been described in one of four dogs kept for long-term evaluation. This animal developed a bladder tumor 3 years after an IORT dose of 30 Gy. This was observed as a filling defect on intravenous pyelography. Microscopic study of the tissue after resection showed a hemangiosarcoma of the bladder within the IORT field. In the same publication two other sarcomas were reported within the IORT field in previously irradiated dogs.

10.2.2 Clinical Results

The largest reported series using IORT in the bladder cancer patients has been from Japan (Matsumoto et al. 1981; 1989). The characteristics of the treatment program tested were preservation of the bladder in combination with a high dose IORT boost of 25–30 Gy and external beam radiotherapy to moderate total doses (30–40 Gy). Other technical aspects of interest were the use of low energy electron beams (4–6 MeV) and the size of the applicators (4, 5, and 6 cm in diameter). In a 10-year period 117 patients were treated. Tumors were generally located at the ureteral orifice, the posterior wall, or the lateral walls, and tumor diameter was less than 3 cm in most cases.

Pathologic tumor stage was Ta, T1, and T2 in 95 cases. The cumulative recurrence rate in these early tumor stages was 29% within 6 years of follow-up. There was a significant difference in recurrence rate between the group with solitary tumors (8%) and the group with multiple tumors (27%). Cystectomy was performed in five cases as rescue treatment for recurrences. The complications related to the treatment program included three cases of flank pain for several days after irradiation, presumably due to acute obstruction of the ureteral orifice, which was included in the irradiation field. No serious late complications were observed except in one patient who had a contracted bladder after 30 Gy IORT and 31.5 Gy external beam irradiation, requiring urinary diversion 12 years later because of progressive bilateral hydronephrosis. Radiation proctitis or other bowel damage was not experienced. Obstruction of the bladder neck or ureteral orifice did not occur. The survival rate for patients with Ta, T1, and T2 tumors is 72%. Thirteen local tumor recurrences have been documented in the period evaluated. No long-term survivors have been seen among T4 patients, but there are some long-term survivors among T3 patients.

In the Western countries occasional long-term survivors have been described, with a functional bladder (Shipley 1989; Martinez and Gunderson 1984).

10.3 Treatment Protocol

Patient selection was based upon pretreatment evaluation that included a complete history and physical examination, a complete blood count, determination of urea nitrogen, serum creatinine, and creatinine clearance, urinalysis, urine cytology, urine culture, and a liver function test. Diagnostic imaging studies included chest radiography, bone scan, excretory urography, and abdominal and pelvic CT. All patients had transurethral sampling of the lesion and bimanual pelvic examination under anesthesia. The tumor size and location, the number of lesions, a gross description of the lesion(s), and the extent of resection were recorded on a separate urologic form. Biopsies were taken from the bed and margins of resections, as well as the areas surrounding the tumor(s). Lesions suspicious for malignancy were resected. Patients with clinical stage T3-T4NxM0, a Karnofsky performance status above 60%, a white blood cell count of more than 3000/mm^3, a platelet count of more than 100 000/mm^3, and creatinine clearance of above 50 cc/min were considered eligible for the protocol.

Pathologic review was performed in all cases before and after cystectomy and the presence of muscle invasion was ascertained. The histologic specimens were examined for typing and grading (G1-4), lymphatic vessel invasion, and the possible presence of residual tumor (PT0/PT+). T status was classified according to the TNM staging system.

The treatment protocol is outlined in Fig. 10.1. The surgical procedure consisted in a midline longitudinal incision to expose the bladder. Both ureters were dissected free over the distal third of their length to ensure that they were excluded from the IORT field. The IORT cone was introduced through the anterior laparotomy incision and the whole collapsed bladder was included in it. The small bowel was mobilized out of the pelvis with fixed retractors. The gantry of the linear accelerator was angulated and the cones were usually beveled (15° or 30°). The rectum was protected with a lead shield in most cases.

External beam radiotherapy started 4 weeks after the first surgical procedure. The treatment consisted in a four-field box technique, including in the target volume the bladder and the pelvic nodal areas. A CT treatment planning system was available in all cases. The daily dose was 2 Gy, and the total dose delivered to the volume was 46 Gy in 5 weeks.

Radical cystectomy was performed 4–6 weeks after external beam radiotherapy. Surgical techniques were uniform for all patients. Male patients underwent radical cystoprostatectomy. An anterior exenteration was carried out in the female patients.

Patients were subsequently pathologically staged. Multiple sections were cut (average: eight) from each cystectomy specimen in order to study the possible presence of tumor cells and other histopathologic features.

Chemotherapy administered in the neoadjuvant group consisted of: cisplatin 15 mg/m^2, 24 h i.v. infusion days 1–3; 5-fluorouracil 1000 mg/m^2 (maximum 1500 mg per 24 h), i.v. infusion days 1–3; doxorubicin 35 mg/m^2, i.v. day 1; hexamethylmelamine 150 mg/m^2, p.o. (maximum dose 200 mg/day) days 8–17.

Three courses of the above-described chemotherapy were given, commencing every 4 weeks. The initial cycle started just after the transurethral resection and the confirmation of invasive bladder cancer. The second chemotherapy course was given after the laparotomy for ureteral diversion, IORT, and lymphadenectomy. The third course started upon the completion of preoperative external beam radiotherapy, 4 weeks before the second surgical intervention for cystectomy.

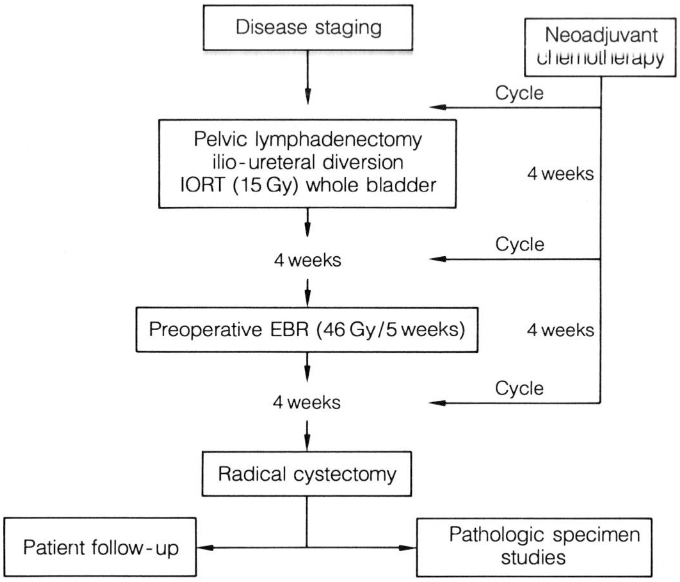

Fig. 10.1. Multidisciplinary treatment program integrating IORT whole bladder boost

10.4 Results

10.4.1 Patient, Tumor, and Treatment Characteristics

This analysis concerns the bladder cancer patients with muscle invasion treated with IORT between September 1984 and December 1989. A total of 23 patients completed the multidisciplinary protocol. Their ages ranged from 44 to 71 years, with a mean of 55 years. There were 22 males and one female. Karnofsky performance status was above 70% in 19 patients. Initial primary tumor stage was classified as T3 in 22 cases and T4 in one.

The radiotherapy characteristics are shown in Table 10.1. All patients received preoperative pelvic irradiation. In 18 cases a single IORT field was used to treat the bladder. Five patients with either advanced local disease or positive pelvic nodes were treated with multiple IORT fields to include the nodal iliac areas in the lateral pelvic wall.

Table 10.1. Patient, tumor, and treatment characteristics in IORT for bladder cancer

	No.	%
Patients	23	100
Age		
Range: 44–71 years		
Mean: 55 years		
Sex		
Male	22	95
Female	1	5
Karnofsky performance status		
>70%	19	82
<70%	4	18
Tumor stage		
T3	22	95
T4	1	5
Radiotherapy		
External beam (preoperative)		
40 Gy	2	9
46 Gy	21	91
IORT[a]		
Cone diameter (cm)		
5–6	10	35
7–8	19	65
Electron energy (MeV)		
6–9	8	27
12–15	18	62
18–20	3	11
Number of fields		
Single	18	78
Multiple	5	22
Total dose (Gy)		
10	9	30
15	20	70

[a] A total of 29 fields treated

The most frequent electron energy employed was 12 MeV; the cone diameter ranged from 5 to 8 cm. The total dose to the bladder was rather homogeneous (15 Gy in 20 patients). In 13 patients neoadjuvant chemotherapy was administered as described in the treatment protocol.

10.4.2 Pathologic Findings After Cystectomy

The cystectomy samples were carefully studied to ascertain the histologic changes induced by 10–15 Gy IORT plus preoperative external beam radiotherapy (46 Gy, with conventional fractionation), with or without neoadjuvant chemotherapy. Several histologic features were present in the bladder at the time of pathologic evaluation, such as mucosal edema (100% of cases), extensive fibrosis (39%), calcifications (21%), findings compatible with a rejected foreign body (44%), and residual tumor cells (26%) (Table 10.2). All patients with residual tumor in the bladder (pT+) were in the group treated upon the initiation of this protocol, and did not receive neoadjuvant chemotherapy.

10.4.3 Patterns of Tumor Recurrence and Survival Data

The median follow-up time for the entire group is 23 months, with follow-up ranging from 3+ to 50+ months. Tumor recurrence has been demonstrated in five patients (two pT+ and three pT0). The site of first tumor recurrence has been distant in all cases (penis, retroperitoneal space, adrenal gland, and bone). In 13 out of 17 patients without evidence of residual tumor in the bladder (pT0), no tumor recurrence has been observed. In three out of six patients with residual tumor in the bladder (pT+), recurrent disease was demonstrated and

Table 10.2. Histologic features in the cystectomy specimens after IORT and preoperative external beam radiotherapy, with or without neoadjuvant chemotherapy

	No. of cases	%
Edema	23	100
Rejected foreign body	10	44
Fibrosis	9	39
Calcification	5	21
Residual tumor cells	6	26

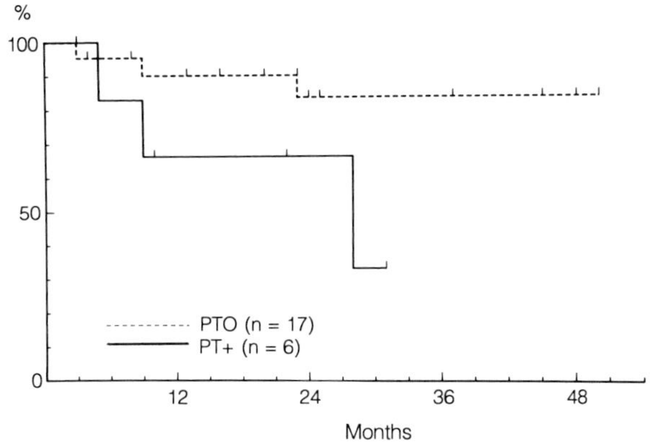

Fig. 10.2. Actuarial survival curves for patients with (pT+) or without (pT0) residual tumor in the bladder following treatment

was the cause of death at 9, 18, and 28 months after IORT. One additional patient died free of malignant disease at 3 months after IORT. Figure 10.2 compares the actuarial survival curves for pT0 and pT+ patients.

10.5 Conclusion

The integration of an IORT boost to the whole bladder in a multidisciplinary protocol combining preoperative irradiation and planned cystectomy, and more recently with the addition of neoadjuvant systemic chemotherapy, has proven to be feasible and well tolerated. The sterilization rate of invasive bladder cancer, confirmed in pathologic studies of the cystectomy specimens, is high (in the range of 70%) and seems to be increased by the addition of neoadjuvant chemotherapy to the treatment program. These findings are of importance with respect to the development of new protocols with the aim of bladder preservation. IORT is a very attractive radiotherapy boosting modality to be considered in the future in this cancer site.

References

Bloom HJG, Hendry WF, Wallace DM, Skeet RG (1982) Treatment of T3 bladder cancer: controlled trial of preoperative radiotherapy and radical cystectomy versus radical radiotherapy. Br J Urol 54: 136–151

Calvo FA, Henriquez I, Santos M et al. (1990) Intraoperative and external beam radiotherapy in invasive bladder cancer: pathological findings following cystectomy. Am J Clin Oncol 13: 101–106

Eapen L, Stewart D, Danjoux C et al. (1989) Intraarterial cisplatin and concurrent radiation for locally advanced bladder cancer. J Clin Oncol 7: 230–235

Hoekstra HJ, Sindelar WF, Kinsella TJ, Mehta DM (1989) Intraoperative radiation therapy-induced sarcomas in dogs. Radiat Res 120: 508–515

Kinsella TJ, Sindelar WF, De Luca AM, Barnes M, Tochner E, Mixon A, Glatstein E (1988) Tolerance of the canine bladder to intraoperative radiation therapy: an experimental study. Int J Radiat Oncol Biol Phys 14: 939–946

Marks LB, Kaufman SD, Prout GR, Heney NM, Griffin PP, Shipley WU (1988) Invasive bladder carcinoma: preliminary report of selective bladder conservation by transurethral surgery, upfront MCV (methotrexate, cisplatin and vinblastine) chemotherapy and pelvic irradiation plus cisplatin. Int J Radiat Oncol Biol Phys 15: 877–883

Martinez A, Gunderson LL (1984) Intraoperative radiation therapy for bladder cancer. Urol Clin North Am 11: 643–698

Matsumoto K (1989) Intraoperative radiation therapy for bladder cancer. In: Dobelbower RR, Abe M (eds) Intraoperative radiation therapy. CRC, Boca Raton, Fl, pp 217–226

Matsumoto K, Kakizoe T, Mikuriya S, Tanaka T, Kondo I, Umegaki Y (1981) Clinical evaluation of intraoperative radiotherapy for carcinoma of the urinary bladder. Cancer 47: 509–513

Montie JE, Straffon RA, Stewart BH (1984) Radical cystectomy without radiation therapy for carcinoma of the bladder. J Urol 131: 477–482

Parsons TJ, Million RR (1988) Planned preoperative irradiation in the management of clinical stage B2-C (T3) bladder carcinoma. Int J Radiat Oncol Biol Phys 4: 797–810

Quilty PM, Duncan W (1986) Primary radical radiotherapy for T3 transitional cell cancer of the bladder: an analysis of survival and control. Int J Radiat Oncol Biol Phys 12: 853–860

Raghavan D (1988) Pre-emptive (neo-adjuvant) intravenous chemotherapy for invasive bladder cancer: review. Br J Urol 61: 1–8

Richie JP, Shipley WU, Yagoda A (1989) Cancer of the bladder. In: De Vita VT, Hellman S, Rosemberg SA (eds) Cancer. Principles and practice of oncology. JB Lippincott, Philadelphia, pp 1008–1022

Shipley WU (1989) Intraoperative radiation therapy for bladder cancer: a review of techniques allowing improved tumor doses and providing high cure rates without the loss of bladder function. In: Dobelbower RR, Abe M (eds) Intraoperative radiation therapy. CRC, Boca Raton, Fl, pp 227–233

Shipley WV, Rose MA, Perrone TL, Mannix CM, Heney NH, Prout GR (1985) Full dose irradiation for patients with invasive bladder carcinoma: clinical and histologic factors prognostic of improved survival. J Urol 134: 679–683

Shipley WU, Kauman DS, Prout GR (1987) Intraoperative radiation therapy in patients with bladder cancer. A review of techniques allowing improved tumor doses and providing high cure rates without loss of the bladder function. Cancer 60: 1485–1488

Skinner DG, Lieskovsky G (1984) Contemporary cystectomy with pelvic node dissection compared to preoperative radiation therapy plus cystectomy in management of invasive bladder cancer. J Urol 131: 1069–1072

Sternberg CN, Yagoda A, Scher HI et al. (1988) M-VAC (methotrexate, vinblastine, doxorrubicin and cisplatin) for advanced transitional cell carcinoma of the urothelium. J Urol 139: 461–469

Van der Werf-Messing BHP, Menon RS, Hop WCJ (1983) Carcinoma of the urinary bladder category T3NxM0 treated by the combination of radium implant and external irradiation: second report. Int J Radiat Oncol Biol Phys 9: 177–180

11 Gynecologic Cancer

FELIPE A. CALVO, DAVID ORTIZ DE URBINA, FERNANDO DE LA FUENTE, MATIAS JURADO, and JOSÉ MARÍA BERIÁN

CONTENTS

11.1	Introduction	79
11.2	Previous Experiences	80
11.2.1	Tissue Tolerance Studies	80
11.2.2	Clinical Results	80
11.3	Treatment Protocols	80
11.3.1	Locally Advanced Primary Tumors	81
11.3.2	Recurrent Pelvic Disease	81
11.4	Analysis of Results	81
11.4.1	General Aspects of the Series	81
11.4.2	Toxicity and Complications	82
11.4.3	Patterns of Relapse	82
11.4.4	Survival Data	83
11.5	Conclusion	83
	References	83

11.1 Introduction

The modern treatment of gynecologic malignancies varies depending on tumor site and histologic type. Combined modality treatment is the treatment of choice in early and intermediate stages of cervical, endometrial, vaginal, and vulvar carcinomas. Locally advanced tumors are approached with radical radiotherapy and/or investigational protocols. Locoregional intensification treatment modalities may play a role in the above-mentioned tumor sites owing to the low risk of distant dissemination of these diseases (HOSKINS et al. 1989). Ovarian cancer has a completely different behavior and treatment. Chemotherapy and debulking surgery are the important components of a radical treatment. The natural tendency of the disease is to metastasize within the abdominal cavity. The integration of radiotherapy programs in the treatment of disease in this site has the disadvantages that the target volume usually includes the complete peritoneal cavity and that only high total doses of radiation will give reasonable local control rates. Normal tissue tolerance commonly limits the possibility to sterilize ovarian cancer with radiotherapy (YOUNG et al. 1989).

Recurrent disease in gynecologic cancer is a major medical problem. In many instances, recurrences are isolated masses within the pelvis that will progress slowly to involve pelvic structures (ureters, bladder, rectum, vessels, nerves, nodes, bones, etc.) and induce medical complications that require palliative procedures (catheters, arterial embolization, pain control, etc.). These patients deserve a great deal of supportive care and medical efforts to ensure the best possible quality of life. Recurrent gynecologic cancer has rarely been approached with second-line radical treatment. Factors such as previous high dose radiotherapy, location and size of the tumor, and normal tissue involvement limit the possibility of rescue surgery. Even if surgery is attempted, these procedures involve risk: extensive organ resections (pelvic exenterations), dissection of major and minor vessels adjacent to or infiltrated by tumor, reconstruction of the urinary and digestive tract, and small bowel manipulation (in cases of previous radiotherapy) carry a high risk of suture dehiscence. Following such types of surgical intervention residual disease may be left in the lateral pelvic walls or other areas of nonresectable pelvic structures.

Intraoperative radiation therapy is an attractive technique for incorporation in the combined treatment of locally advanced primary tumors in which known residual disease or high risk margins for microscopic tumor involvement are left following surgical resection, usually in the parametrial space (Fig. 11.1). In an adjuvant setting, IORT might yield the highest local control rates, which is the aim of this technique. In recurrent cases, the results that may be expected from the incorporation of IORT in disease management will at the least be as good as those obtained with surgery alone. However, any increase in pelvic tumor control

FELIPE A. CALVO, Dr., Director and Consultant, DAVID ORTIZ DE URBINA, Dr., Radiotherapy Division, Department of Oncology, FERNANDO DE LA FUENTE, Dr., Consultant, MATIAS JURADO, Dr., Department of Gynecology, JOSÉ M. BERIÁN, Dr., Consultant, Department of Urology, Clinica Universitaria de Navarra, 31080 Pamplona, Spain

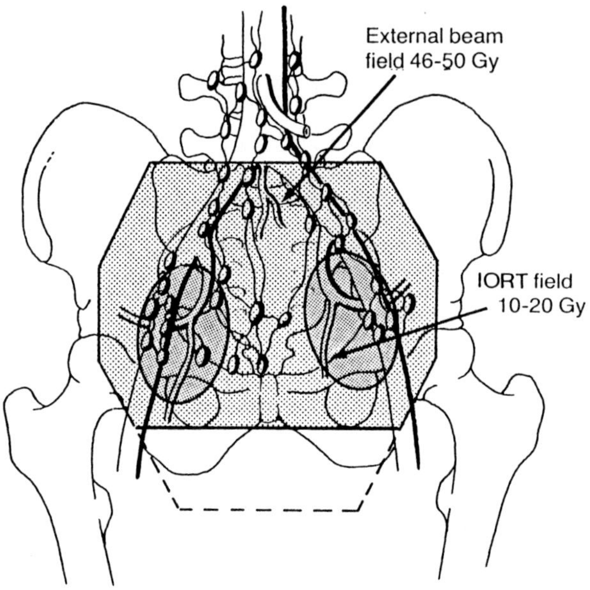

Fig. 11.1. Diagram illustrating the integration of IORT for the treatment of the lateral pelvic walls following resection

rates that is obtained will be at the expense of an increase in normal tissue damage and complications due to the fact that a substantial proportion of these patients will have been treated previously with radical irradiation. The possible role of IORT in the treatment of ovarian cancer is at present unknown, but it is probably limited to those cases in which there is small pelvic or abdominal tumor persistence or recurrence after systemic treatment.

11.2 Previous Experiences

11.2.1 Tissue Tolerance Studies

The target of IORT during gynecologic cancer surgery is the pelvic walls and the presacral space. Organs and structures such as the rectum, bladder, and ureters are either not present at the time of IORT (pelvic exenterations) or can be easily excluded from the IORT cone by mobilization. Therefore the fixed structures that cannot be protected in many instances are nerves, vessels, and bone. In cases involving technical difficulties during tumor resection the IORT field will include vascular sutures (generally the iliac vein). A number of studies in animal models have analyzed the tolerance of these tissues and structures to either high single doses of IORT (Sindelar et al. 1983; Kinsella et al. 1985; Hoekstra et al. 1985) or high single doses of IORT combined with fractionated external beam radiotherapy (Hoopes et al. 1987; Le Coteur et al. 1989; Powers et al. 1989); the results can be reasonably extrapolated to the clinical setting.

An interesting line of experimental basic research would be to analyze the tissue tolerance of nerves, vessels, and bone to treatment with high dose external beam radiotherapy (46–50 Gy) followed by a rest period (10–20 months) and then treatment with escalating single doses of IORT. Such studies would provide a model to follow in most cases of recurrent tumor located in pelvic organs previously treated with high dose external beam radiotherapy.

11.2.2 Clinical Results

The available clinical data regarding the use of IORT for the treatment of gynecologic malignancies were obtained in phase I–II trials in small series of patients treated for recurrences or locally advanced primary tumors, with a variety of histologies (Delgado et al. 1984; Calkins et al. 1985; Terashima et al. 1980). It is interesting to note that IORT was employed in early studies (Goldson et al. 1978) to treat para-aortic nodes (with or without pelvic side wall fields) in gynecologic cancer. A recent review of this experience showed that of 19 patients treated (16 of whom had squamous cell carcinomas and three, adenocarcinomas), 11 had positive para-aortic nodes while eight were negative. Median survival time was 17 and 33 months respectively. Treatment-related complications were arterial hemorrhage (2), pelvic abscess (1), neuropathy (2), ureteral obstruction (1), vena cava laceration (2), leg edema (3), and prolonged ileus (2). Vascular complications were seen after 25 Gy IORT and 45 Gy external beam radiotherapy (Goldson et al. 1989).

11.3 Treatment Protocols

Intraoperative radiation therapy has been integrated in our institution in the multidisciplinary management of gynecologic tumors. Two different treatment programs have been employed: (a) IORT in combination with rescue surgery for recurrent disease following previous radiotherapy; (b) IORT in combination with surgery and planned pre- or postoperative pelvic irradiation, with or without simultaneous continuous infusion chemotherapy.

11.3.1 Locally Advanced Primary Tumors

Intraoperative radiation therapy (15–20 Gy) has been used as a boost to areas of residual disease or areas at high risk for tumor recurrence following surgical resection. Planned pre- or postoperative pelvic irradiation (46–50 Gy) was always used, and simultaneous continuous infusion of cisplatin 40 mg/m^2 plus 5-fluorouracil 1000 mg/m^2 was given over the first 4 and the last 4 days of the external beam course.

11.3.2 Recurrent Pelvic Disease

This category includes patients with pelvic recurrences following any surgical treatment and a full course of external beam radiotherapy. The treatment protocol included exploratory laparotomy, tumor resection if possible, or tumor exposure, and IORT (15–20 Gy) in the areas of residual disease. External beam radiotherapy was always omitted.

11.4 Analysis of Results

11.4.1 General Aspects of the Series

This analysis includes all patients at our institution who were treated with IORT and had a histologically confirmed diagnosis of gynecologic malignancy during the period 1984–1989.

Table 11.1. Patient characteristics ($n = 27$)

	No.	%
Age		
Range: 15–72 years		
Median: 52 years		
Karnofsky performance status		
< 70%	19	70
> 70%	8	30
Disease status		
Recurrent[a]	19	70
Primary	8	30
Initial pelvic pain	23	85

[a] Including patients with previous surgery and/or radical radiotherapy

11.4.1.1 Patient Characteristics

The total number of patients treated was 27. Their ages ranged from 15 to 72 years, with a median of 52 years. A high proportion of the patients (70%) had a low Karnofsky performance status. In 19 cases the disease was recurrent following previous treatments (surgery, radiotherapy, and/or chemotherapy), while eight new cases were diagnosed and staged in our institution (Table 11.1).

11.4.1.2 Tumor Characteristics

The series comprised 17 cervical, five endometrial, four ovarian, and one vulvar carcinomas. Histologic investigation revealed 17 squamous cell carcinomas, nine adenocarcinomas, and one mixed müllerian sarcoma. Tumor stages in newly diagnosed patients were: IIB 4, III 2, and IV 2 (Table 11.2).

11.4.1.3 Treatment Characteristics

The types of surgical intervention performed were as follows: four laparotomies with no resection and tumor exposure, three anterior exenterations, 11 total exenterations, and nine hysterectomies plus nodal dissection. Postsurgical residual tumor was judged to be macroscopic in 20 cases and microscopic in seven (Table 11.3). Pelvic irradiation was carried out preoperatively in 21 cases and postoperatively in six external beam radiotherapy was given in all cases. Neoadjuvant simultaneous chemotherapy was administered in 12 cases, post-

Table 11.2. Tumor characteristics

	No.	%
Location		
Cervix	17	63
Endometrium	5	18
Ovary	4	14
Vulva	1	3
Histology		
Squamous cell ca.	17	63
Adenocarcinoma	9	33
Mixed müllerian	1	4
Stage		
Pelvic recurrence	19	40
IIB	4	15
IIIA-B	2	7
IVA-B	2	7

Table 11.3. Surgical treatment characteristics

	No.	%
Type of operation		
Tumor exposure (no resection)	4	15
Anterior exenteration	3	11
Total exenteration	11	41
Hysterectomy plus nodal dissection	9	33
Postsurgical residual disease		
Gross residual disease	20	74
Microscopic residual disease	7	26

operative adjuvant chemotherapy in one case, and palliative chemotherapy in six cases (Table 11.4).

11.4.2 Toxicity and Complications

Various acute but reversible complications were seen – postoperative pelvic bleeding (2), prolonged ileus (5), perineal wound infection (4), iliac vein thrombosis (1), and lymphocele (1). Severe complications observed in the postoperative period were dehiscence of intestinal sutures (3) and vesicovaginal fistula (1). These severe complications diagnosed in the postoperative period were seen in three patients with recurrences in a previously irradiated pelvis and in one patient with no previous treatment.

Long-term sequelae observed were pelvic pain (10), paresthesia and lower extremity weakness (5), ureteral stricture requiring catheter placement (2), minor unilateral lymphedema (1), urinary incontinence (1), and rectosigmoid fibrosis with slight stenosis (2) (Table 11.5).

Table 11.4. Radiotherapy and chemotherapy characteristics

	No. of patients
Pelvic recurrences	
No previous radiotherapy	4
Previous radiotherapy	15
40–50 Gy	9
>50 Gy	6
Primary tumors	
Preoperative (46–50 Gy)[a]	6
Postoperative (46–50 Gy)	2
Neoadjuvant simultaneous chemotherapy	12
Adjuvant postoperative chemotherapy	1
Palliative chemotherapy	6
No chemotherapy	8

[a] Includes two cases with simultaneous neoadjuvant chemotherapy

Table 11.5. Toxicity and complications

	No. of patients
Acute complications	
Pelvic bleeding	2
Wound infection	4
Prolonged ileus	5
Suture dehiscence (intestinal)	3
Vesicovaginal fistula	1
Iliac vein thrombosis	1
Lymphocele	1
Late sequelae	
Pelvic pain	10
Lower extremity neuropathy	5
Ureteral stricture	2
Rectosigmoid fibrosis	2
Lymphedema	1
Urinary incontinence	1

11.4.2.1 Pelvic Pain

The development of pelvic pain in patients with gynecologic cancer treated with IORT merits further comment. Pelvic pain is present at the time of treatment evaluation in some patients with locally advanced or recurrent gynecologic cancer and is related to the involvement of the sciatic nerve. However, IORT in the range of single doses that have been employed can induce pelvic pain in patients treated for pelvic tumors (Shaw et al. 1987, 1990). In our series, pelvic pain was present at the initial evaluation in 23 patients, and improved slightly after IORT in half of them. Only two patients with no pelvic pain at presentation developed this symptom following IORT. In the follow-up of all patients with pelvic pain and neurologic symptomatology related to IORT, five cases progressed to lower extremity paresthesia. No irreversible motor loss was seen.

11.4.3 Patterns of Relapse

Local failure in this tumor site is defined as any tumor recurrence within the pelvis. In our experience it is difficult to assess accurately in pelvic IORT the status of the treated field. In gynecologic cancer, one should distinguish between central failures (vaginal) and lateral pelvic failures. In our series ten local failures were seen among the 27 patients treated: five in patients with recurrent disease and five in patients with primary disease. The median length of follow-up for the entire series was 12+ months. Combined local and dis-

Table 11.6. Patterns of recurrence in relation to disease status

Disease status	No.	LF	LF + DM	DM
Recurrent[a]	15	4	1	3
Primary	12	5	–	1
Total	27	9	1	4

Abbreviations: LF, local failure; DM, distant metastasis
[a] Patients with previous radiotherapy

tant relapse was diagnosed in one patient and distant dissemination as the only site of failure in four (Table 11.6).

11.4.4 Survival Data

Median survival time has been 15 months for the entire group: it has been 14 months in patients with recurrent disease while in patients with primary disease it has not yet been reached. Follow-up time since IORT has ranged from 1+ to 38 months. At the time of this analysis nine patients are alive and free of tumor, four are alive with progressive disease, one has died free of tumor, and 13 have died with tumor progression (ten in the recurrent group and three in primary disease group). Actuarial survival curves are shown in Fig. 11.2.

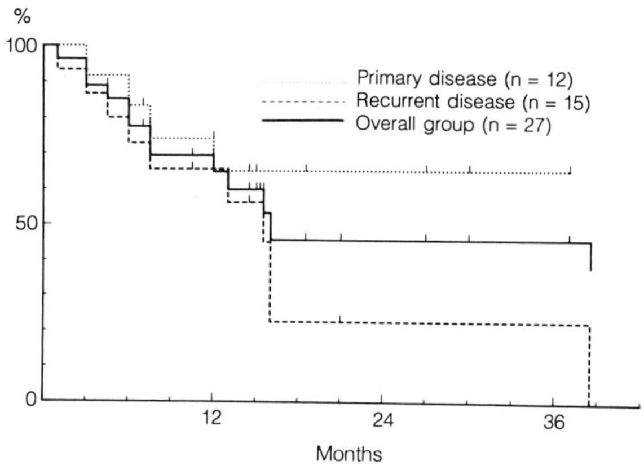

Fig. 11.2 Actuarial survival curves for gynecologic patients treated with IORT

11.5 Conclusion

Gynecologic cancer comprises a miscellaneous group of tumor sites and histologies in which treatment with IORT has been explored in heterogeneous protocols. From our own experience and previous data, it is difficult to draw any firm conclusions regarding the use of IORT. The pelvis is the most difficult area in which to perform IORT. Recurrent pelvic disease requires laborious surgery with a high risk of morbidity and even mortality in the pre- and postoperative period. The decision to operate on such patients should be made on an individualized basis. Even when performing large tissue resections with adequate normal tissue margins and removing all the intrapelvic contents, these patients are still at high risk for local recurrence. With this in mind, it does not seem the most appropriate disease entity for exploration of IORT with curative intent, but IORT may still remain a means of promoting local tumor control in highly selected cases. Sophisticated boosting techniques such as brachytherapy have a role to play and are most indicated in early and intermediate tumor stages. This is probably the appropriate time for IORT as well. There is a lack of information on normal tissue tolerance after high dose external beam irradiation (with or without brachytherapy boost) with a rest period of several months and then high single doses of IORT. Understanding and cooperation on the part of gynecologic oncologists would be of great value in the development of IORT trials in this area of oncology.

References

Abe M, Takahashi M (1981) Intraoperative radiotherapy: the Japanese experience. Int J Radiat Oncol Biol Phys 7: 863–868

Calkins A, Stehman F, Lester S et al. (1985) A prospective trial of intraoperative radiation therapy in recurrent pelvic malignancy. Proc Am Soc Clin Oncol 4: 275

Delgado G, Goldson AL, Ashaveri E et al. (1984) Intraoperative radiation in the treatment of advanced cervical cancer. Obstet Gynecol 63: 246–252

Goldson AL, Delgado G, Hill LT (1978) Intraoperative radiation of the para-aortic nodes in cancer of the uterine cervix. Obstet Gynecol 52: 713–717

Goldson AL, Delgado G, Ashayeri E, Petrilli ES (1989) Intraoperative electron beam radiation therapy for gynecological malignancies. In: Dobelbower RR, Abe M (eds) Intraoperative radiation therapy. CRC, Boca Raton, Fl, pp 247–263

Hoekstra HJ, Kinsella TJ, Maher M et al. (1985) Treatment complications related to intraoperative radiotherapy. Proc Am Soc Clin Oncol 4: 254

Hoopes PJ, Gillette EL, Withrow SJ (1987) Intraoperative irradiation of the canine abdominal aorta and vena cava. Int J Radiat Oncol Biol Phys 13: 715–722

Hoskins WJ, Perez CA, Young RC (1989) Gynecologic tumors. In: De Vita VT, Hellman S, Rosenberg SA (eds) Cancer. Principles and practice of oncology, vol 1, 3rd edn. JB Lippincott, Philadelphia, pp 1099–1150

Kinsella TJ, Sindelar WF, De Luca AM, Terrill R (1985) Tolerance of peripheral nerve to intraoperative radiotherapy (IORT) clinical and experimental studies. Int J Radiat Oncol Biol Phys 11: 1579–1585

Le Coteur RA, Gillette EL, Powers BE et al. (1989) Peripheral neuropathies following experimental intraoperative radiation therapy (IORT). Int J Radiat Oncol Biol Phys 17: 583–590

Powers BE, Gillette EL, McChesney SL et al. (1989) Bone necrosis and tumor induction following experimental intraoperative irradiation. Int J Radiat Oncol Biol Phys 17: 559–567

Shaw EG, Gunderson LL, Martin JK et al. (1987) Toxicity and results of intraoperative radiation therapy for primary unresectable and recurrent pelvic malignancies. Am J Clin Oncol 10: 105

Shaw EG, Gunderson LL, Martin JK et al. (1990) Peripheral nerve and ureteral tolerance to intraoperative radiation therapy: clinical and dose response analysis. Radiother Oncol 18: 247–255

Sindelar WF, Kinsella TJ, Tepper J, Travis EL, Rosenberg SA (1983) Experimental and clinical studies with intraoperative radiotherapy. Surg Obstet Gynecol 157: 205–219

Terashima H, Takayama K, Jimi S, Watanabe Y (1980) Intraoperative irradiation for advanced ovarian cancer. Nippon Gan Chiryo Gakkai Shi 15: 329–333

Young RC, Fuks Z, Hoskins WJ (1989) Cancer of the ovary. In: De Vita VT, Hellman S, Rosenberg SA (eds) Cancer. Principles and practice of oncology, vol 1, 3rd edn. JB Lippincott, Philadelphia, pp 1162–1191

12 Retroperitoneal and Other Central Soft Tissue Sarcomas

Felipe A. Calvo, Oscar Abuchaibe, José María Serra, José Mariá Berián, and José Cañadell

CONTENTS

12.1	Introduction	85
12.2	Previous Experiences	85
12.2.1	Tissue Tolerance Studies	85
12.2.2	Clinical Studies	86
12.3	Treatment Protocol	88
12.4	Results	88
12.4.1	Patient, Tumor, and Treatment Characteristics	88
12.4.2	Patterns of Recurrence	89
12.4.3	Toxicity and Complications	89
12.4.4	Outcome and Survival Data	89
12.5	Conclusion	89
	References	90

12.1 Introduction

Soft tissue sarcomas involving anatomic zones other than the extremities are rare and have generally been treated by surgical resection. Since the production of evidence that radiation therapy can increase local control in soft tissue sarcomas of the extremities (Rosenberg et al. 1982), radiotherapy has been used more frequently postoperatively. Surgical resection of soft tissue sarcomas of the retroperitoneum, head and neck, trunk, or pelvis will achieve clear margins in only a few cases. Success in this respect depends not only on tumor size and technical skills but also on the anatomic site involved by tumor.

The ability of sarcomas to progress distantly through the pseudocapsule, through fascia and neurovascular structures, should also be considered. Radiation therapy techniques have been optimized over recent decades and high energy photons, electron beams, CT treatment planning, and brachytherapy are tools that have contributed to the delivery of high doses of radiation in carefully designed radiotherapy programs. (Pilepich and Antoniades 1987). Nevertheless, the final outcome in patients with soft tissue sarcomas located in central anatomic areas is poorer than that in patients with lesions of the extremities. The rates of local tumor control are lower, in general due to marginal recurrences, and in the case of tumors in certain locations, such as intra-abdominal lesions, the risk of distant recurrences seems to be increased (Chang et al. 1989). Chemotherapy is being investigated, but an optimal regime in this subgroup of soft tissue sarcoma patients still has to be defined.

Intraoperative radiation therapy has been utilized more actively in intra-abdominal soft tissue sarcomas than in lesions of the extremities (Dobelbower and Abe 1989). The technique offers an attractive sophisticated radiation boost to tumor bed areas, with protection of many of the normal, uninvolved tissues surrounding the lesion. This approach allows reduction of the external beam total doses to a tolerable level, and accurate definition of the area at risk for recurrence. The technique requires close cooperation between surgeons and radiation oncologists because these lesions are usually large at the time of diagnosis or recurrent following previous surgery, and because adequate exposure of the tumor bed may be extremely difficult. In extra-abdominal soft tissue sarcomas (head and neck, trunk, etc.) the technique is much simpler and the most relevant questions are which nerves should be included in the IORT field and how much residual disease is left after surgery, factors of importance to the dose selection process.

12.2 Previous Experiences

12.2.1 Tissue Tolerance Studies

The tolerance of retroperitoneal structures to IORT has been investigated in animal models

---

Felipe A. Calvo, Dr., Director and Consultant, Oscar Abuchaibe, Dr., Radiotherapy Division, Department of Oncology, José M. Serra, Dr., Consultant, Department of Reconstructive and Plastic Surgery, José M. Berián, Dr., Consultant, Department of Urology, José Cañadell, Dr., Consultant, Department of Orthopedic Surgery and Traumatology, Clinica Universitaria de Navarra, 31080 Pamplona, Spain

(Sindelar et al. 1982). In a dog model, a treatment port including partially the kidney, ureter, aorta, vena cava, and retroperitoneal soft tissues received single doses of high energy electrons (11 MeV) of 20, 30, 40, and 50 Gy. No complications or histologic changes occurred in any animal given doses of 20 Gy, with a follow-up in excess of 18 months. At 30 Gy one case of ureteral obstruction was observed. In the 40 Gy group, mild vascular fibrosis of the aorta and vena cava occurred, together with ureteral fibrosis. All animals that received 50 Gy died of radiation-related complications.

In the clinical setting, patients will be treated not only with a high single dose of electron beam but also with external beam radiotherapy, which makes it important to analyze radiobiologic studies using both radiation modalities together. Moreover, radical surgery for large retropertoneal sarcomas will in many cases involve ipsilateral nephrectomy, leaving as possible dose-limiting structures to IORT the aorta, the posterior abdominal wall, nerves, the vena cava on the left side, and to some extent the vertebral bodies (Figs. 12.1, 12.2). The tissue changes induced by escalating doses of IORT and 50 Gy conventional fractionated external beam radiotherapy have

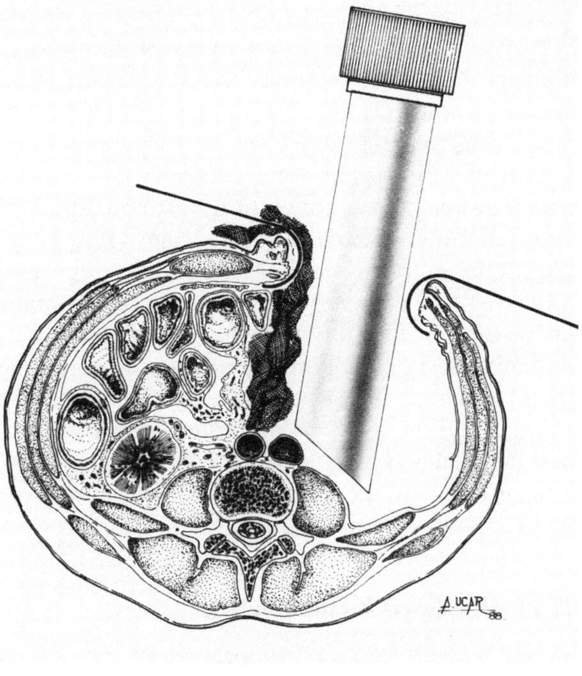

Fig. 12.1. Illustration of the technique for IORT following resection of a retroperitoneal sarcoma (nephrectomy was performed)

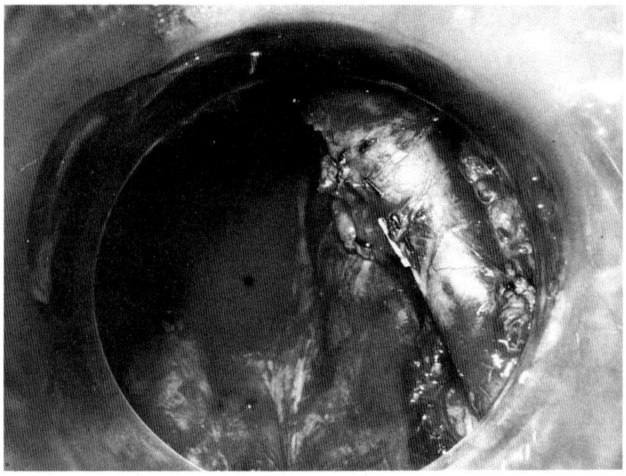

Fig. 12.2. View of the treatment field through the IORT cone following resection of a retroperitoneal sarcoma

been extensively investigated. Tissue tolerance has been studied in bone (Powers et al. 1989b), muscle (Powers et al. 1989a), and large vessels (Gillette et al. 1988). The results suggested that 10–15 Gy is the IORT boost dose range that is relatively safe in combination with 50 Gy external irradiation. Higher IORT doses (20, 25, or 30 Gy) led to more pronounced tissue changes; extrapolated into clinical practice this would mean that risk is increased. The ureter and peripheral nerves were confirmed to be two important dose-sensitive structures.

12.2.2 Clinical Studies

Data regarding the use of IORT in the treatment of retroperitoneal soft tissue sarcomas have been reported from several Western institutions (Dobelbower and Abe 1989). In the Massachusetts General Hospital series (Tepper et al. 1989), 13 patients with retroperitoneal sarcomas and two with sarcomas located in the chest cavity were treated with preoperative external beam irradiation and 15–20 Gy IORT followed by surgical resection. The 5-year survival rate was 39%, with an actuarial local control rate of 80% (three local failures). One patient with a primary tumor of the chest cavity developed fatal pneumonitis. The local control rates compared favorably with the results obtained without IORT in the same institution (Tepper et al. 1984).

At the Mayo Clinic (Gunderson et al. 1989) some intra-abdominal sarcomas approached by

IORT surgery and external beam radiotherapy were reported. In six cases disease was recurrent and in two primary cases the lesions were not amenable to radical surgery. All patients (four) with disease progression developed distant metastases after treatment. A larger analysis has been reported by the same group, pertaining to the period April 1981 to February 1988 (GUNDERSON et al. 1988). In 19 evaluable patients with soft tissue sarcomas of the abdomen and pelvis, a combined treatment program was implemented including resection, 10, 15, 17.5, or 20 Gy IORT boost to the tumor bed, and 45–60 Gy external beam irradiation. Ten patients had recurrent disease at the time of IORT. The patterns of failure showed three local recurrences and six distant progressions (including one case of peritoneal seeding). One local failure was rescued with hemipelvectomy. Survival analysis showed 14 patients to be alive, with ten free of disease (follow-up ranged from 13 to 67 months). Significant complications related to IORT occurred in five patients: nerve (1), wound (2), urologic (1), and fibrosis (1). The authors concluded that the aggressive treatment approach appeared to be promising in view of the high rate of local tumor control, and that even selected patients with locally recurrent disease might benefit.

At the Rush-Presbyterian-St. Luke's Medical Center (KIEL et al. 1989) four patients with retroperitoneal sarcomas treated with IORT have been reported. Local control was achieved in two patients with primary disease. Local and marginal recurrences were detected in the remaining two patients. At the time of analysis three patients were alive, two free of disease at 10 and 41 months, and one with disease at 21 months. The review of the experience at the Medical College of Ohio (DOBELBOWER et al. 1989) showed that seven patients with a diagnosis of central sarcomas had been treated with IORT over a 4-year period. Tumor locations were: chest wall (3), pelvis (2), retroperitoneum (1), and paravertebral (1). Five had recurrent disease following previous treatment. Four received additional external beam irradiation after surgery and IORT. Three patients were alive and free of disease at the time of publication, with follow-up ranging from 7 to 35 months. The remaining four patients developed local recurrences. One patient with a pelvic primary developed ipsilateral extremity neuropathy.

Preliminary results of a randomized study of adjuvant radiation therapy (including IORT) in resectable retroperitoneal soft tissue sarcomas in adults have been reported by the National Cancer Institute (USA) group (KINSELLA et al. 1988). Over a period of 5 years, 35 patients were randomized to receive surgery plus high dose external beam radiotherapy (50–55 Gy) or surgery, IORT (20 Gy), and a moderate dose of external beam radiotherapy (35–40 Gy). Of 87 patients evaluated for this treatment program, 15 were treated with IORT with a tumor stage distribution as follows: stage II – one, stage III – four, and stage IV – 10. Among the 20 patients treated in the standard arm, five were stage II, seven stage III, and eight stage IV. The minimum follow-up at the time of publication was 15 months and there was no significant difference in overall survival or disease-free survival in the two treatment groups. The median disease-free survival time was 38 months for the standard treatment group compared with 20 months for the experimental (IORT) group. At 5 years, approximately 40% of patients were alive and 20% were disease free. There was no difference in locoregional control, the assessment of which included any tumor recurrence in the retroperitoneum and/or peritoneal cavity. The median time to local progression was 38 months in the standard treatment group, while it had not been reached in the IORT group. There appeared to be a certain improvement in "in field" control with the combination of IORT and low dose external beam radiotherapy, although it was not statistically significant. The treatment complication rate in the whole group was 63%, with no significant difference between the IORT and control arms. Acute radiation enteritis was observed in 12 patients in the standard group and in one patient in the IORT group; in the follow-up period seven patients in the standard group and two in the IORT group developed chronic enteritis.

Four patients in the IORT group and one in the standard group developed reversible neuropathy involving the femoral-sciatic-sacral nerve plexus (in the patient in the standard group this was surgically induced). Other complications that occurred with similar frequency in both groups were infections, ureteral obstruction, gastrointestinal hemorrhage, cardiopulmonary complications, and vascular insufficiency. The final comments made by the authors regarding the study results were that IORT plus reduced external beam total dose can be delivered with less morbidity than high dose external irradiation alone, but that there is no significant improvement in long-term survival and freedom from relapse.

12.3 Treatment Protocol

Patients with soft tissue sarcomas located in central anatomic zones have been treated in our institute with the best surgical resection possible, IORT to the tumor bed area (12–20 Gy), and fractionated external beam radiotherapy (45–50 Gy). Chemotherapy is recommended in patients with high cellular grade sarcoma. In patients with recurrent disease after high dose external beam radiotherapy, reirradiation was omitted and IORT was the only radiation technique employed.

12.4 Results

This report is a detailed update of the experience previously published (Calvo et al. 1989).

12.4.1 Patient, Tumor, and Treatment Characteristics

Twenty-four patients treated over a 5-year period are available for analysis. Ten were males and 14, females. Their ages ranged from 7 to 77 years (median 45 years). Karnofsky performance status was equal or superior to 70% in all patients. Disease at the time of evaluation for IORT was recurrent in 12 cases, and in 7 of these 12 cases the recurrence was in a previously irradiated area (Table 12.1).

There was a wide variety of histologic subtypes. The most frequent diagnoses were malignant

Table 12.1. Characteristics of patients (n = 24) treated with IORT for central and retroperitoneal soft tissue sarcomas

	No. of patients
Sex	
Male	10
Female	14
Age	
Mean: 45 years	
Range: 7–77 years	
Karnofsky performance status	
Mean: 80%	
Range: 70%–100%	
Disease status	
Recurrent	12
Primary	12

Table 12.2. Characteristics of the central soft tissue sarcomas treated by IORT

	No. of patients
Histology	
Malignant fibrous histiocytoma	5
Liposarcoma	3
Rhabdomyosarcoma	4
Leiomyosarcoma	1
Hemangiopericytoma	3
Synovial cell sarcoma	1
Schwannosarcoma	1
Pleomorphic sarcoma	2
Dermatofibrosarcoma	1
Grade	
I	4
II	8
III	12
Stage	
I	6
II	3
III	4
IVa	11
Location	
Head and neck	3
Trunk	7
Retroperitoneum	6
Pelvis	5
Gluteus	3

Table 12.3. Radiotherapy characteristics of the treatment program

	No. of patients
IORT	
Cone diameter (cm)[a]	
5–7	9
8–10	14
12–15	3
Number of fields[a]	
Single	10
Multiple	14
Electron energy (MeV)[a]	
6–9	11
12–15	11
18–20	3
Total dose[a] (Gy)	
10	10
15	10
20	6
25	1
External beam radiotherapy (Gy)	
40	6
45–50	11
Not given	7

[a] Thirty-eight fields used

Table 12.4. Patterns of recurrence in patients with central soft tissue sarcomas treated with IORT ($n = 24$)

Sarcoma site	Local failure	Local failure + distant metastasis	Distant metastasis
Head and neck	–	1	–
Trunk	–	2	2[a]
Retroperitoneum	2[a,b]	2	–
Pelvis	–	1	–
Gluteus	3[b]	–	–
Total	5 (21%)	6 (25%)	2 (8%)

[a] Lung and para-aortic nodes
[b] Local failures rescued with further surgery and IORT (one patient in each site)

fibrous histiocytoma, rhabdomyosarcoma, and liposarcoma. There were 12 cases of high cellular grade sarcomas. Locally advanced tumor stages III and IVa were established in 15 cases. Tumor locations were: head and neck (3), trunk (7), retroperitoneum (6), pelvis (5), and gluteus (3) (Table 12.2).

Surgery did not achieve clear surgical margins in any patients but microscopic residual disease was assumed in 11 patients. A total of 38 IORT fields were used to cover the areas at risk for residual disease. Ten procedures required a single field to encompass the desired volume, while 14 procedures were performed with multiple IORT fields. Cone diameter ranged from 5 to 15 cm, but the most frequently used sizes were 8, 9, and 10 cm. The electron energy selected was 6–9 MeV in the 11 cases with microscopic residual disease postsurgically (11) and 12–20 Gy in those cases with gross residual disease. The single IORT doses most frequently used were 10 and 15 Gy. External beam radiotherapy was added in 17 cases, with doses ranging from 40 to 50 Gy (Table 12.3).

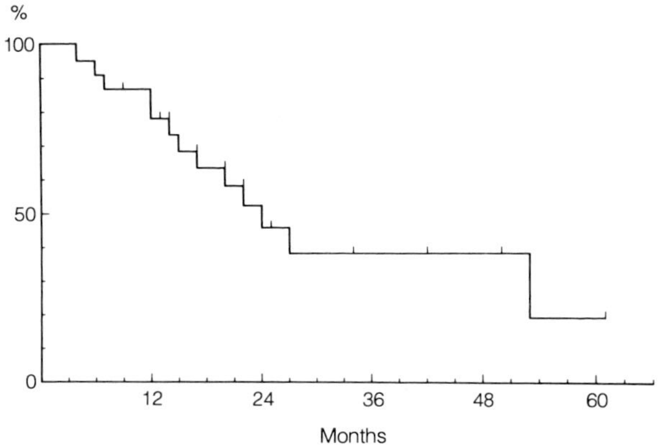

Fig. 12.3. Actuarial survival curve for central soft tissue sarcoma patients treated with IORT

12.4.2 Patterns of Recurrence

Local failure alone was observed in five cases (two retroperitoneal and three gluteal tumors). Two of these patients were rescued with surgery. Combined local and systemic failures were seen in six patients, and distant dissemination as the only site of tumor progression was detected in two patients. In 8 of the 11 local recurrences a careful analysis of the area of tumor recurrence suggested that the disease progressed marginally to the IORT field (Table 12.4).

12.4.3 Toxicity and Complications

Some IORT-related complications were identified in this group, including: myclopathy (1), reversible peripheral neuropathy (2), transient pneumonitis with long-term lung fibrosis (1), and vertebral collapse with sclerotic bone changes (1).

12.4.4 Outcome and Survival Data

The actuarial survival curve is shown in Fig. 12.3. At the time of analysis 11 patients are alive and 13 have died, all from progressive neoplastic disease. The median survival time for the entire group was 23 months, with a follow-up range for surviving patients from 8+ to 61+ months. There are survivors in each tumor location (Table 12.5).

12.5 Conclusion

The local control rate in central soft tissue sarcomas is modest in our experience. None of the

Table 12.5. Outcome after IORT for central soft tissue sarcomas

Sarcoma site	No. of patients	Local control	Patient status Alive/dead
Head and neck	3	2	1/2
Trunk	7	5	2/5
Retroperitoneum	6	3[a]	2/4
Pelvis	5	4	4/1
Gluteus	3	1a	2/1
Total	24	15 (63%)	11/13

[a] Patients rescued with further surgery and IORT

treated patients would have been cured with surgery alone, owing to the lack of tumor-free normal tissue margins at the time of resection. There are survivors among both the recurrent and the primary tumor patients, and in each tumor location. As in previous clinical series, it was not uncommon to find recurrences at the margins of the IORT and/or external beam radiotherapy fields, which suggests that the area considered at risk for residual disease is not adequately evaluated. The phase III trial reported in retroperitoneal sarcomas serves as a point of reference for the design of future studies (Kinsella et al. 1988).

References

Calvo FA, Abuchaibe O, Escude L et al. (1989) Intraoperative radiotherapy in the multidisciplinary management of soft tissue sarcomas. Ann Radiol 32: 489–492

Chang AE, Rosenberg SA, Glatstein EJ, Antman KH (1989) Sarcomas of soft tissues. In: De Vita VT, Hellman S, Rosenberg SA (eds) Principles and practice of oncology, 3rd edn. JB Lippincott, Philadelphia, pp 1345–1398

Dobelbower RR, Abe M (eds) (1989) Intraoperative radiation therapy. CRC, Boca Raton, Fl

Dobelbower RR, Eltaki A, Bronn DG (1989) Intraoperative radiation therapy: the Medical College of Ohio experience. In: Dobelbower RR, Abe M (eds) Intraoperative radiation therapy. CRC, Boca Raton, Fl, pp 313–354

Gillette EL, Powers BE, McChesney SL et al. (1988) Response of aorta and branch arteries to experimental intraoperative irradiation. Int J Radiat Oncol Biol Phys 15 [Suppl 1]: 202

Gunderson LL, Nagorney DM, Macilrath DC et al. (1988) External beam and intraoperative electron irradiation for soft tissue sarcomas. Int J Radiat Oncol Biol Phys 15 [Suppl 1]: 184

Gunderson LL, Martin JK, Nagorney DM et al. (1989) Mayo Clinic experience with intraoperative and external beam irradiation with or without resection. In: Dobelbower RR, Abe M (eds) Intraoperative radiation therapy. CRC, Boca Raton, Fl, pp 287–298

Kiel K, Kramer T, Roseman DL (1989) The Rush-Presbyterian-St. Luke's Medical Center experience with intraoperative radiation therapy. In: Dobelbower RR, Abe M (eds) Intraoperative radiation therapy. CRC, Boca Raton, Fl, pp 299–312

Kinsella TJ, Sindelar WF, Lack E et al. (1988) Preliminary results of a randomized study of adjuvant radiation therapy in resectable adult retroperitoneal soft tissue sarcomas. J Clin Oncol 6: 18–25

Le Coteur RA, Gillette EL, Powers BE et al. (1989) Peripheral neuropathies following experimental intraoperative radiation therapy (IORT). Int J Radiat Oncol Biol Phys 17: 583–590

Pilepich MV, Antoniades J (1987) Soft tissue sarcomas. In: Perez CA, Brady LW (eds) Principles and practice of radiation oncology. JB Lippincott, Philadelphia, pp 1182–1198

Powers BE, Gillette EL, McChesney SL et al. (1989a) Muscle injury following experimental intraoperative irradiation. Int J Radiat Oncol Biol Phys 17 [Suppl 1]: 246

Powers BE, Gillette EL, McChesney SL et al. (1989b) Bone necrosis and tumor induction following experimental intraoperative irradiation. Int J Radiat Oncol Biol Phys 17: 559–567

Rosenberg SA, Tepper JE, Glatstein E et al. (1982) The treatment of soft tissue sarcomas of the extremities. Prospective randomized evaluations of (1) limb-sparing surgery plus radiation therapy compared with amputation and (2) the role of adjuvant chemotherapy. Ann Surg 196: 305–314

Sindelar WF, Tepper J, Travis EL, Terrill R (1982) Tolerance of retroperitoneal structures to intraoperative irradiation. Ann Surg 96: 601–608

Tepper JE, Suit H, Wood WC, Proppe KH, Harmon D, McNulty P (1984) Radiation therapy of retroperitoneal soft tissue sarcomas. Int J Radiat Oncol Biol Phys 10: 825–830

Tepper JE, Shipley WU, Wood WC et al. (1989) Intraoperative radiation therapy at the Massachusetts General Hospital. In: Dobelbower RR, Abe M (eds) Intraoperative radiation therapy. CRC, Boca Raton, Fl, pp 279–286

13 Soft Tissue Sarcomas of the Extremities

Felipe A. Calvo, David Ortiz de Urbina, José L. Beguiristain, Santiago Amillo, and José Cañadell

CONTENTS

13.1	Introduction	91
13.2	Previous Experiences	91
13.2.1	Tissue Tolerance Studies	91
13.2.2	Clinical Results	92
13.3	Treatment Protocol	92
13.3.1	Surgery	92
13.3.2	IORT	92
13.3.3	External Beam Radiotherapy	93
13.3.4	Chemotherapy	94
13.4	Analysis of Results	94
13.4.1	General Aspects of the Series	94
13.4.2	Toxicity and Complications	95
13.4.3	Patterns of Relapse	95
13.4.4	Survival Data	96
13.5	Conclusion	96
	References	96

13.1 Introduction

The procurement of high local control rates using a combined modality approach and preservation of functional extremities represent two challenges in the treatment of soft tissue sarcomas located in the extremities (Eilber et al. 1980). Systemic therapy is an important component of the treatment of high grade sarcomas and/or large primary tumors, in which the development of distant metastases still makes it difficult to achieve definitive cure of the disease. Randomized trials have established that survival is not compromised by extremity preservation treatment, and adequate combination of surgery and radiotherapy yields survival data as good as those achieved by amputation (Rosenberg et al. 1982). Local recurrences occur in 20%–25% of cases treated by conventional surgical resection and external beam radiotherapy (Suit et al. 1985). IORT is an alternative boosting technique that has rarely been explored in a systematic fashion in soft tissue sarcomas of the extremities (Dobelbower and Abe 1989).

Use of IORT in tumor bed areas in the extremities following tumor resection has only minor advantages from the point of view of normal tissue protection. The skin is the sole structure always to be protected. Occasionally portions of the nerves can be dissected so as to mobilize and protect them from the radiation beam. Despite this technical limitation, IORT might exploit other mechanisms to improve the therapeutic index of combined treatment; for example, it is possible to achieve excellent delimitation of the area of residual disease or the area at high risk of local recurrence at the time of surgical removal of the tumor, and a high single dose of radiotherapy is delivered directly to such areas.

13.2 Previous Experiences

13.2.1 Tissue Tolerance Studies

In soft tissue sarcomas of the extremities, IORT fields will include normal tissues like muscle, nerves, vessels, and occasionally bone. Tissue tolerance to high single doses of electrons has been studied in animal models (Kinsella and Sindelar 1985). Peripheral nerve has proven to be a dose-limiting structure in IORT trials with severe clinical consequences if the dose is excessive (Kinsella et al. 1985). Animal data showed a threshold dose for peripheral neuropathy when only IORT was given (damage occurred with single doses over 15 Gy) (Kinsella et al. 1988). A recent report analyzed the development of peripheral neuropathy in dogs using escalated doses of IORT only or IORT combined with external beam irradiation (50 Gy). Electrophysiologic ab-

---

Felipe A. Calvo, Dr., Director and Consultant, David Ortiz de Urbina, Dr., Radiotherapy Division, Department of Oncology, José L. Beguiristain, Dr., Consultant, Santiago Amillo, Dr., José Cañadell, Dr., Consultant, Department of Orthopedic Surgery and Traumatology, Clinica Universitaria de Navarra, 31080 Pamplona, Spain normalities were found in one out of five and two out of five animals treated with 15 Gy IORT plus 50 Gy external irradiation and 15 Gy IORT alone respectively. Neurologic lesions increased in incidence with higher doses. A combination of histologic changes were observed, including loss of axons and myelin, increased connective tissue in the endoneural, perineural, and epineural areas, and necrosis and hyalinization of the media of small arteries and arterioles. The onset of peripheral neuropathy was similar in the groups of animals treated (usually between 6 and 18 months), and no recovery from nerve damage was observed (LE COTEUR et al. 1989).

The same group of researchers has studied the effects of IORT alone or in combination with external beam radiotherapy in muscle (POWERS et al. 1989a), bone (POWERS et al. 1989b), and major arteries (GILLETTE et al. 1988). Various degrees of histologic changes were seen in those tissues.

In summary, it can be suggested that when tissues like muscle, bone, nerves, and vessels have to be included in the IORT field, such as in some cases of soft tissue sarcomas of the extremities, the dose selected for the IORT component of the treatment has to be a compromise in the range of 10–15 Gy, in an effort to reduce the risk of long-term complications.

13.2.2 Clinical Results

Few clinical data are available from previous reports on the use of IORT in the combined management of soft tissue sarcomas of the extremities. A 73% local control rate was obtained with IORT alone in a series of 29 patients (ABE and TAKAHASHI, 1981), and a positive attitude to the continued investigation of this modality has been recommended (TEPPER et al. 1989).

13.3 Treatment Protocol

The treatment protocol employed in the Clinica Universitaria de Navarra in patients with localized soft tissue sarcomas of the extremities has remained the same over the past 5 years. Local treatment has consisted in the combination of maximal surgical resection with preservation of the involved extremity, IORT boost to the tumor bed and/or residual disease (10–20 Gy), and external beam irradiation (46–50 Gy). Chemotherapy has been given to patients with high grade (II–III) histologies and rhabdomyosarcoma.

13.3.1 Surgery

Although the rationale of surgery for soft tissue sarcomas has been uniform (i.e., removal of as much macroscopic tumor as possible), the incision size and location have varied depending upon the morphologic characteristics of the tumor. The following points are of relevance to the adequate planning of the treatment procedure in sarcomas of the extremities:

- The incision should extend 2–3 cm above and below the tumor mass. This will aid skin protection and ensure that the tumor bed has a margin of normal tissues around it.
- The staging diagnostic imaging procedures have to be directed towards the relationship between the tumor and major vessels and nerves. If these structures are reasonably distant from the tumor, shielding or dissection for mobilization from the IORT field can be planned before surgery.
- The posterior margin of the tumor is usually the area at higher risk for residual disease, and biopsy sampling of this area will help to determine whether there is residual tumor after resection. In general in sarcoma surgery the positioning of the patient and the direction of the incision are important, and the anterior and lateral limits of the tumor can be dissected leaving a certain margin of normal tissue. The posterior part of the tumor is an uncomfortable area for surgeons: the neovascularization is visualized with more difficulty and the resection limit tends to be close to the pseudocapsule of the tumor.

13.3.2 IORT

Following removal of the tumor it is important to examine the macroscopic aspect of the surgical specimen, analyzing carefully the size and marginal areas. The tumor bed is defined as the area possibly in contact with the tumor, which includes the posterior and lateral surrounding tissues. These tissues have to be exposed to the electron beam like an "opened book," retracting muscles

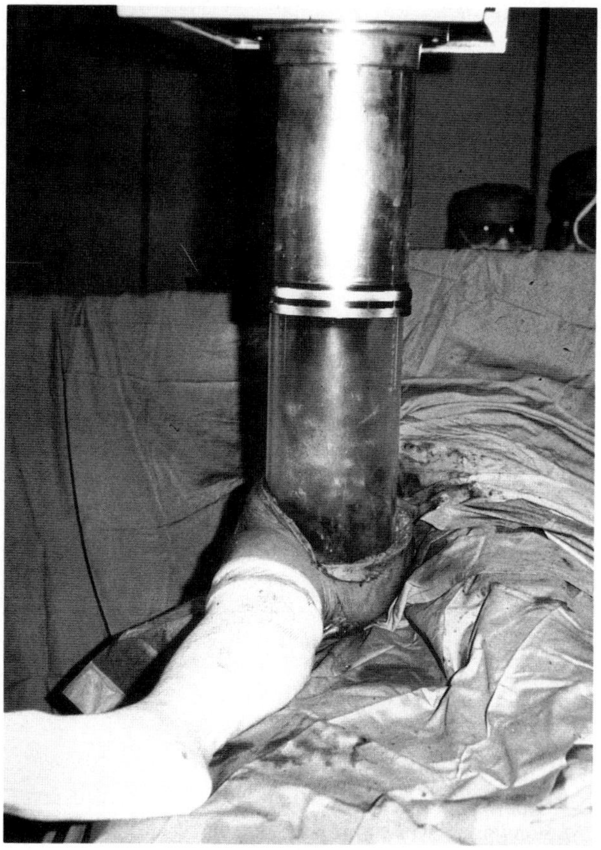

Fig. 13.1. Example of an IORT procedure for a large liposarcoma of the thigh

in such a way as to present to the electron beam the area at risk. Careful hemostasis is always recommended to avoid bleeding during IORT and a "build-up effect." The electron energy is selected in accordance with the thickness of the tissue to be treated. If the nerves are to be shielded, lead shields will be needed to cover the area. Gantry angulation and cone size differ from one procedure to another depending upon the characteristics of the surgical approach (Figs. 13.1, 13.2). In general, the use of multiple adjacent IORT fields is not recommended. Sometimes, however, an additional small field is needed to cover adequately the area of risk in cases of sarcoma of the upper thigh extending to the iliac fossa. In general the direction of this beam will be different from the original one treating the tumor bed. Measurements to avoid overlapping are not needed.

13.3.3 External Beam Radiotherapy

The treatment technique consists in a conventional approach using 6 MV photons, bolus material in the incision scar, and a large target volume with normal tissue margins, leaving a corridor of skin and soft tissues to avoid lymphedema. Other technical details are the use of parallel opposed fields,

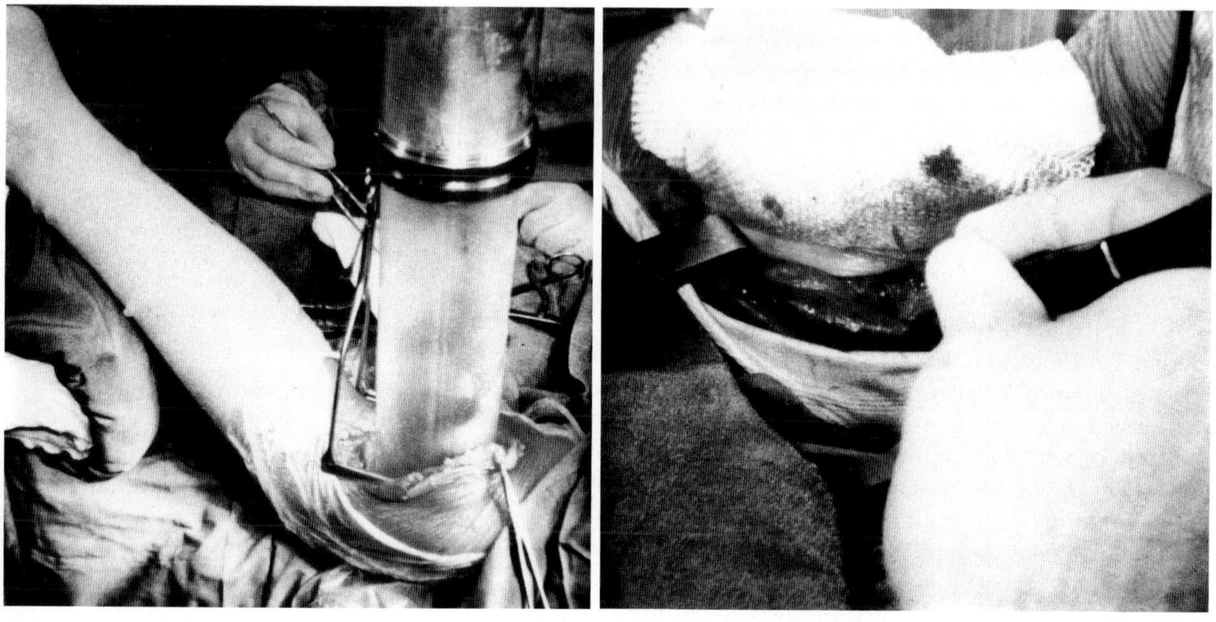

b

Fig. 13.2a,b. Popliteal nerve mobilized outside the IORT cone in a synovial sarcoma of the lower extremity

CT planning and dosimetry, and use of external beam radiotherapy with delivery of 2 Gy per daily fraction, five times a week, reaching total doses in the range of 46–50 Gy. No cone-down fields are used (IORT is the boosting technique), and occasionally mixed photon and electron beams have been employed for peripherally located lesions.

13.3.4 Chemotherapy

Chemotherapy has been administered to patients with rhabdomyosarcoma and high grade tumors. Neoadjuvant chemotherapy was considered for patients with large tumors, recurrences following previous treatments, and/or rhabdomyosarcoma. A uniform regime of Adriamycin, dacarbazine, ifosfamide, cisplatin, and amphotericin B was investigated as a phase II protocol (Campbell et al. 1988). Neoadjuvant treatment consisted in three cycles, and adjuvant treatment, in six postoperative courses. All patients showed some degree of objective tumor response to neoadjuvant chemotherapy.

13.4 Analysis of Results

13.4.1 General Aspects of the Series

This analysis includes patients with localized soft tissue sarcomas of the extremities treated at the Clinica Universitaria de Navarra between 1984 and 1989. Three patients receiving IORT were excluded due to the presence of distant metastases at the time of surgery.

13.4.1.1 Patient Characteristics

The total number of patients available for analysis is 19. Their ages ranged from 11 to 71 years, with a median of 36 years. Eight were males and 11, females. Karnofsky performance status was equal to or less that 70% in five and above 70% in 14. At the time of reevaluation for IORT, three patients had local recurrences subsequent to previous radical external beam radiotherapy; two have had prolonged chemotherapy for a local recurrence after radical surgery alone. In total 12 cases in this series were considered recurrent disease at the time of entering the IORT program (Table 13.1).

Table 13.1. Patient (n = 19) characteristics

	No.
Age	
Median: 36 years	
Range: 11–71 years	
Sex	
Male	8
Female	11
Karnofsky performance status	
≤70%	5
>70%	14
Previous treatment	
Surgery	14
Radiotherapy	3
Chemotherapy	2
Disease status at diagnosis	
Primary	7
Recurrent	12

Table 13.2. Tumor characteristics

	No.
Histology	
Liposarcoma	5
Fibrosarcoma	4
Malignant fibrous histiocytoma	4
Rhabdomyosarcoma	3
Hemangiopericytoma	1
Leiomyosarcoma	1
Synovial sarcoma	1
Location	
Upper extremity	4
Lower extremity	15
Grade	
I	5
II	7
III	7

13.4.1.2 Tumor Characteristics

Table 13.2 shows the histologic subtypes, cellular grades, and tumor locations. Liposarcomas were low grade, and the lower extremity was the predominant location.

13.4.1.3 Treatment Characteristics

Gross residual disease was present at the completion of surgery in two patients. In the remaining 17 cases surgery achieved apparently complete resection. The IORT technique included the use of 25 fields, 13 single and six multiple. Cone diameter was 8 cm or more in 18 fields. The most frequent electron energies selected were 9 and 12 MeV.

Table 13.3. Treatment characteristics

	No.
Surgery	
Complete resection	17
Incomplete resection	2
IORT	
Number of fields	
Single field	13
Multiple fields	6
Cone diameter (cm)[a]	
5–7	7
8–10	11
12–15	7
Electron energy (MeV)[a]	
6–9	9
12–15	15
18–20	1
Total dose (Gy)	
10	4
15	12
20	9
External beam radiotherapy	
46–50 Gy	18
Not done	1
Chemotherapy	
Neoadjuvant + adjuvant	9
Adjuvant	3

[a] The total number of IORT fields treated was 25

The initial protocol was designed to deliver 20 Gy IORT, but as soon as neuropathy was observed in some of the early cases, the IORT doses were decreased to 10–15 Gy. External beam radiotherapy (46–50 Gy) was given to 18 patients. Two of the three recurrences in a previously irradiated area were retreated (in one case a musculocutaneous flap was used to cover the area). Chemotherapy was used in a neoadjuvant and adjuvant fashion in nine patients, and in three as an adjuvant treatment (Table 13.3).

13.4.2 Toxicity and Complications

In the immediate postoperative period a few minor and reversible complications occurred after IORT. There were some severe complications in the long-term follow-up of these patients. Severe irreversible peripheral neuropathy was seen in three patients, one patient developed a femoral fracture while free of disease progression, one patient had a venous thrombosis which recovered with medical treatment, and six patients had a moderate degree of soft tissue fibrosis in the area treated with the external beam irradiation (Table 13.4).

Table 13.4. Toxicity and complications

	No.
Postsurgical period	
Fever	1
Delayed wound healing	1
Wound infection	1
Thrombophlebitis	2
Long-term events	
Severe peripheral neuropathy	3
Femoral bone fracture	1
Vein thrombosis	1
Soft tissue fibrosis	6

13.4.2.1 Peripheral Neuropathy

The three patients with peripheral neuropathy are still alive and free of disease progression. One of these patients had a rhabdomyosarcoma, one a hemangiopericytoma, and one a liposarcoma. Sensory and subsequent motor loss were experienced by the patients at 10, 11, and 14 months after IORT. All received 20 Gy IORT plus 46 Gy external beam radiotherapy. Two of these patients had had tumor recurrences following previous surgery. Pain and dysesthesia were reported by the patients 1–2 months before the onset of loss of neurologic function. Amputation of the damaged extremity has not to date been necessary in any of the patients.

13.4.3 Patterns of Relapse

The median follow-up time for the entire series is 24+ months. Two local recurrences have been diagnosed; three patients have developed distant metastases (lung). One of the local recurrences occurred in a patient with a malignant fibrous histiocytoma located anterior to the tibia and treated with 15 Gy IORT and 46 Gy external beam radiotherapy. The recurrence was established at 32 months after completion of treatment. The second local recurrence was in a patient retreated with surgery and IORT in a previously irradiated area. A single dose of 20 Gy IORT was administered, and macroscopic residual disease was left after surgery. The relapse or persistence was histologically documented 7 months after IORT.

13.4.3.1 Salvage Treatment

The patient with a primary tumor and recurrence had an amputation, and is alive and free of disease at 42 months' follow-up. The other local recurrence was in the inguinal area. The patient refused surgical intervention and is presently receiving systemic chemotherapy. Patients with lung metastases (three cases) have been treated with thoracotomy; one is alive and apparently free of tumor progression and two have died from progressive disease in spite of second- and third-line chemotherapy.

13.4.4 Survival Data

The survival data at present show 14 patients alive and free of disease, one alive with disease, and four dead; two patients died with disease progression and two died while free of disease (one from sepsis during chemotherapy aplasia, and one from cardiomyopathy). The actuarial survival curve is shown in Fig. 13.3.

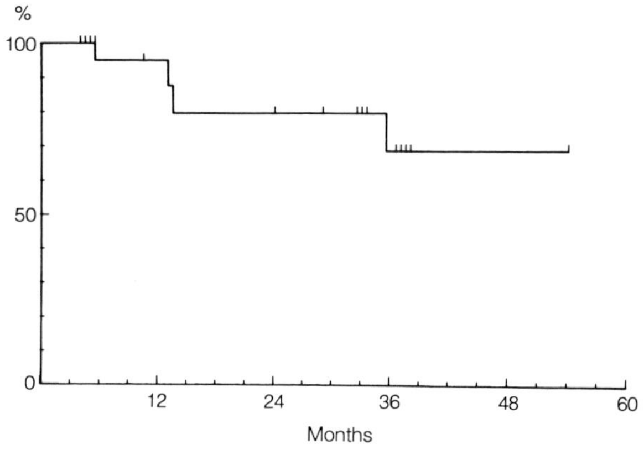

Fig. 13.3. Actuarial survival curve for patients treated with IORT for soft tissue sarcomas of the extremities

13.4.4.1 Preservation of Extremities

In the 19 patients treated, one amputation has been performed due to a local recurrence. Four extremities have a poor functional status; in three there is total motor and sensory loss and in one, a progressive local recurrence. The upper extremities treated are fully functional. In the lower extremities the functional status is good even in cases with wide muscular removal and long-term soft tissue fibrosis.

13.5 Conclusion

The use of IORT with surgery and external beam radiotherapy appears of interest in the local treatment of soft tissue sarcomas of the extremities. Local control rates are encouraging. A word of caution is necessary regarding the selection of the total IORT dose for future trials. In our initial experience three out of seven patients treated with 20 Gy IORT developed severe neuropathy. In the remaining four patients treated with 20 Gy, the nerves were not included in the field (three cases) or were shielded (one case). All patients treated with 10 Gy IORT plus external beam radiotherapy had the nerves in the field and did not develop neuropathy. In the 15 Gy IORT group (nine cases), four had the nerves treated without subsequent neuropathy, but there was one local recurrence. In summary, it appears that 10–15 Gy might be the dose range that leads to high local control rates with minor long-term complications. A further interesting observation in our series is that out of 14 patients with previous surgery, seven had macroscopic tumor resection and came to our institution for a second opinion. Reexploration and IORT were recommended, and in all cases residual disease was confirmed pathologically in the second surgical procedure. As a final comment on IORT technique in this tumor site, it should be mentioned that for large lesions, large IORT cones should be selected. This implies that the nerves and vessels will not be protected. In these cases, a compromise in the total IORT dose has to be reached. Vascular bypass can be of help in some cases (one was performed in our series), but even in such situations the nerves will rarely be movable for retraction outside the radiation beam.

References

Abe M, Takahashi M (1981) Intraoperative radiotherapy: the Japanese experience. Int J Radiat Oncol Biol Phys 7: 863–868

Campbell W, Beloqui O, Herranz P et al. (1988) Ifosfamide (IFX), doxorubicin (ADM), dacarbazine (DTIC), and amphotericin B (AMB) in metastatic soft tissue sarcoma. Proc Am Assoc Cancer Res 29: 222

Dobelbower RR, Abe M (1989) Intraoperative radiation therapy. CRC, Boca Raton, Fl

Eilber FR, Mirra JJ, Grant TT et al. (1980) Is amputation necessary for sarcomas? A seven year experience with limb salvage. Ann Surg 192: 431–438

Gillette EL, Powers BE, McChesney SL et al. (1988) Response of aorta and branch arteries to experimental intraoperative irradiation. Int J Radiat Oncol Biol Phys 15 [Suppl 1]: 202

Kinsella TJ, Sindelar WF (1985) Intraoperative radiotherapy. In: De Vita VT, Hellman S, Rosenberg SA (eds) Cancer. Principles and practice of oncology. JB Lippincott, Philadelphia, pp 2293–2304
Kinsella TJ, Sindelar WF, De Luca AM et al. (1985) Tolerance of peripheral nerve to intraoperative radiotherapy (IORT): clinical and experimental studies. Int J Radiat Oncol Biol Phys 11: 1579–1585
Kinsella TJ, Sindelar WF, De Luca AM (1988) Threshold dose for peripheral nerve injury following intraoperative radiotherapy (IORT) in a large animal model. Int J Radiat Oncol Biol Phys 15 [Suppl 1]: 205
Le Coteur RA, Gillette EL, Powers BE et al. (1989) Peripheral neuropathies following experimental intraoperative radiation therapy (IORT). Int J Radiat Oncol Biol Phys 17: 583–590
Powers BE, Gillette EL, McChesney SL et al. (1989a) Muscle injury following experimental intraoperative irradiation. Int J Radiat Oncol Biol Phys 17 [Suppl 1]: 246
Powers BE, Gillette EL, McChesney SL et al. (1989b) Bone necrosis and tumor induction following experimental intraoperative irradiation. Int J Radiat Oncol Biol Phys 17: 559–567
Rosenberg SA, Tepper JE, Glatstein E et al. (1982) The treatment of soft tissue sarcomas of the extremities. Prospective randomized evaluations of (1) limb-sparing surgery plus radiation therapy compared with amputation and (2) the role of adjuvant chemotherapy. Ann Surg 196: 305–314
Suit HD (1983) Patterns of failure after treatment of sarcoma of soft tissue by radical surgery or by conservative surgery and radiation. Cancer Treat Symp 2: 241–246
Suit HD, Mankin HJ, Woods WE et al. (1985) Radiation and surgery in the treatment of primary sarcoma of the soft tissue. Pre-operative, intra-operative and postoperative. Cancer 55: 2659–2667
Tepper JE, Wood WC, Suit HD (1989) Intraoperative radiation therapy of soft tissue sarcomas. In: Dobelbower RR, Abe M (eds) Intraoperative radiation therapy. CRC, Boca Raton, Fl, pp 275–278

14 Ewing's Sarcoma

Felipe A. Calvo, Oscar Abuchaibe, Carlos Villas, José Cañadell, and Luis Sierrasesúmaga

CONTENTS

14.1 Introduction . . . 99
14.2 Previous Experiences . . . 99
14.3 Treatment Protocol . . . 100
14.3.1 Primary Disease . . . 100
14.3.2 Recurrent Disease . . . 100
14.4 Results . . . 100
14.4.1 Patient, Tumor, and Treatment Characteristics . . . 100
14.4.2 Toxicity and Complications . . . 101
14.4.3 Patterns of Disease Recurrence . . . 101
14.4.4 Outcome and Survival Data . . . 101
14.5 Conclusion . . . 101
References . . . 102

14.1 Introduction

Ewing's sarcoma is a malignant disease that requires multimodal treatment to obtain high cure rates (Malwer et al. 1989). Radiation therapy is an important component of the treatment of the primary lesion. The reported rates of local control attributed to radiation therapy vary widely (Halperin et al. 1989). Tumor volume and the site of the primary tumor have been related to major differences in local tumor control. Thus isolated local recurrences have been reported in 15% of patients with lesions of the extremities, in 47% with rib primaries, and in 69% with pelvic tumors (Brown et al. 1987). The rate of local persistence/tumor recurrence, as evaluated by clinical and autopsy findings, was reported by Tepper et al. (1980) to be 35%, 25%, and 7% in patients treated with primary radiation therapy for central, proximal extremity, and distal extremity lesions respectively (Tepper et al. 1980). Overall rates of local tumor control with radiotherapy are in the region of 90% for lesions less than 8 cm in maximum diameter, and 70% for those more than 8 cm in maximum diameter (Marcus and Million 1984).

Surgical resection has attracted increasing interest in the management of Ewing's sarcoma (Rosen 1978). Several reports have described improvement in local control and survival with the addition of surgery (Bacci et al. 1982; Brown et al. 1987; Jurgens et al. 1988; Sailder et al. 1988). With reference to the clinical data available, it has to be noted that surgery in Ewing's sarcoma has been used in selected patients with positive prognostic factors such as lesions of the extremities, small tumor volumes, and a good response to chemotherapy. The use of surgery in the management of Ewing's sarcoma patients simultaneously provides an opportunity to consider the use of IORT as a radiation boosting modality in areas of residual disease or at high risk of tumor recurrence.

The conceptual advantages of the inclusion of IORT in the local treatment of Ewing's sarcoma include the accuracy with which the area at high risk for recurrence can be identified at the time of surgery, the ability to protect normal uninvolved tissues when lesions are located in central anatomic zones (pelvic bones, vertebra, etc.), and the possibility of reducing the total external beam radiotherapy dose.

14.2 Previous Experiences

The use of IORT has been reported in only a few cases. At the National Cancer Institute (USA) IORT was used in some patients with pelvic primary lesions (Stea et al. 1987), but no conclusions can be drawn from this limited experience. Tolerance studies in normals tissue involving the use of surgery and IORT boost alone or in combination with external beam radiotherapy

Felipe A. Calvo, Dr., Director and Consultant, Oscar Abuchaibe, Dr., Radiotherapy Division, Department of Oncology, Carlos Villas, Dr., Consultant, José Cañadell, Dr., Consultant, Department of Orthopedic Surgery and Traumatology, Luis Sierrasesúmaga, Dr., Consultant, Pediatric Oncology Unit, Department of Pediatrics, Clinica Universitaria de Navarra, 31080 Pamplona, Spain have suggested that the acceptable tolerated doses in peripheral nerves, muscle, large vessels, and bone are in the range of 15–20 Gy (KINSELLA et al. 1985, 1988; LE COTEUR et al. 1989; POWERS et al. 1989a, 1989b; GILLETTE et al. 1988; KINSELLA et al. 1988).

14.3 Treatment Protocol

The initial experience in our institution with IORT in the multidisciplinary management of Ewing's sarcoma was gained in patients with recurrent disease, in whom surgery and IORT were employed to try to salvage a local failure following previous chemotherapy and external beam radiotherapy. This approach showed a high local control rate with acceptable clinical tolerance. IORT was later included in the treatment of those Ewing sarcoma patients undergoing surgical resection. The treatment program varied from primary to recurrent cases, as will be explained below.

14.3.1 Primary Disease

Patients with the diagnosis of Ewing's sarcoma who had not been previously treated and who had no evidence of systemic disease were treated with preoperative fractionated irradiation (40–45 Gy) to the primary tumor field plus a margin of normal tissues, concomitantly with the initiation of systemic chemotherapy. The chemotherapy regimen has been previously described (SIERRASESUMAGA 1989). Between 4 and 6 weeks after the completion of radiotherapy, patients were considered for surgery and an IORT boost of 10–15 Gy was added to the residual tumor or tumor bed area. Patients received adjuvant chemotherapy for 10–12 months.

In this group of patients with primary disease, there were three cases of protocol violation that have to be described in order to explain the types of toxicity later found. Two patients with large primary tumors in the lower extremities received a single dose of external beam radiotherapy of 10 Gy the day before surgery (flash technique); the remaining radiotherapy was given postoperatively in a conventional program. One additional patient underwent surgical resection after 60 Gy of radical irradiation. Apart from these protocol violations the primary disease group was consistently treated with moderate preoperative irradiation and IORT boost (10–15 Gy).

14.3.2 Recurrent Disease

In patients with local recurrences in previously irradiated areas attempts at salvage were made by means of surgical resection and an IORT boost of 20 Gy to the residual tumor or tumor bed area. At the same time, systemic chemotherapy was employed once more in an effort to prevent the development of metastatic disease.

14.4 Results

14.4.1 Patient, Tumor, and Treatment Characteristics

Over a 5-year period, 20 patients were treated with IORT for Ewing's sarcoma. Their ages ranged from 4 to 32 years, with a median age of 13 years. There were 13 males and seven females. Karnofsky performance status was above 70% in 13 patients. There were six patients with recurrent disease (previously treated with chemotherapy and radiotherapy), of whom three had evidence of metastatic disease.

Tumor size was measured using CT imaging and the overall tumor volume was calculated to be more than 300 cm^3 in 11 cases (six primary tumors and five cases of recurrent disease). The involved bones were femur (3), fibula (3), tibia (5), pelvis (3), vertebrae (2), radius (2), and humerus (1); one case had an extraosseous location.

Following surgery macroscopic residual disease was left in seven cases (including four recurrent tumors); complete resection was performed in 13 cases. External beam radiotherapy was omitted in the recurrent cases except in two patients who received low dose reirradiation.

The IORT technique included the use of a single field in all patients with primary disease, and of the patients with recurrences, only two with recurrent large tumors required multiple fields to encompass the target volume. The electron energies selected were in most cases in the lower spectrum of the available range with our linear accelerator: 6, 9, or 12 MeV. The majority of procedures were performed with IORT cones of 8, 9, 10, and 12 cm in diameter (Table 14.1).

Table 14.1. Tumor and treatment characteristics in patients with Ewing's sarcoma ($n = 20$)

	Primary	Recurrent
Tumor		
Size (volume)		
$\leq 300\,cm^3$	6	5
$>300\,cm^3$	8	1
Involved bone		
Femur	2	1
Fibula	2	1
Tibia	4	1
Pelvis	1	2
Vertebrae	2	–
Radius	1	1
Humerus	1	–
Extraosseous	1	–
Treatment		
Surgery		
Macroscopic residue	3	4
Microscopic residue	11	2
Radiotherapy		
Preoperative	8	1
Postoperative	3	1
Pre- + postoperative	2	1
Not done	1	3
IORT		
Cone diameter (cm)		
6–8	4	5
9–12	9	3
15	1	–
Electron energy (MeV)		
6–9	11	5
12–20	3	3
Total dose		
10	8	1
15	5	6
20	1	1
Number of fields		
Single	14	4
Multiple	–	2

14.4.2 Toxicity and Complications

This analysis is focused on the description of local observations in the area of surgery and radiotherapy. Patients had several infectious and aplasic episodes as a result of the adjuvant chemotherapy program. In three patients delayed wound healing and severe soft tissue necrosis were seen in the follow-up period. These three cases comprised the two treated with high dose flash (10 Gy) preoperative radiotherapy and one additional case that was operated on after radical external beam radiotherapy (60 Gy). Two patients recovered from the soft tissue damage after repair of their lesions with myocutaneous flap. The remaining patient required amputation after failure of conservative management.

Table 14.2. Patterns of disease recurrence in Ewing's sarcoma patients treated with IORT

Disease status	Local failure	Local failure + distant metastasis	Distant metastasis
Primary	–	1	3
Recurrent	–	–	2
Total	–	1	5

In seven patients a minor to moderate degree of soft tissue fibrosis was evident during the follow-up period.

14.4.3 Patterns of Disease Recurrence

At the time of this review only one local recurrence had been identified among the 20 patients treated. This was in a patient with a vertebral primary (C4) who developed a neck mass and multiple brain metastases 8 months following IORT. Five patients have developed distant progression of the disease (three in previously known metastatic sites) (Table 14.2).

14.4.4 Outcome and Survival Data

The median follow-up time of the entire series is 26 months (range, 2–65+ months); the median survival time has not been reached. As an anecdotal detail it has to be mentioned that the longest IORT survivor in our institution is among this group of patients with Ewing's sarcoma: The first patient treated with IORT was a 22-year-old with the diagnosis of Ewing's sarcoma involving the T10 vertebral body. The patient was treated in September 1984 and up to the present has no evidence of disease.

Actuarial analysis of overall survival for the entire group and for primary versus recurrent disease is shown in Figs. 14.1 and 14.2, respectively.

14.5 Conclusion

In this exceptional series exploring IORT in a pediatric radiosensitive tumor such as Ewing's sarcoma, the initial local control rate is encouraging. Surgery is now being considered more frequently in the overall management of this disease, and

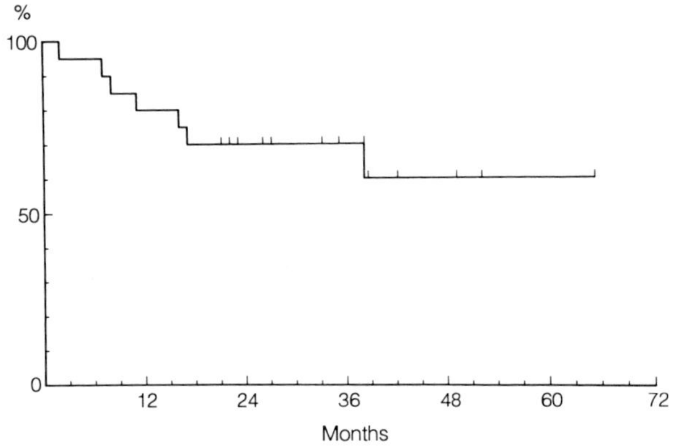

Fig. 14.1. Actuarial survival curve for the entire series of Ewing's sarcoma patients treated with IORT

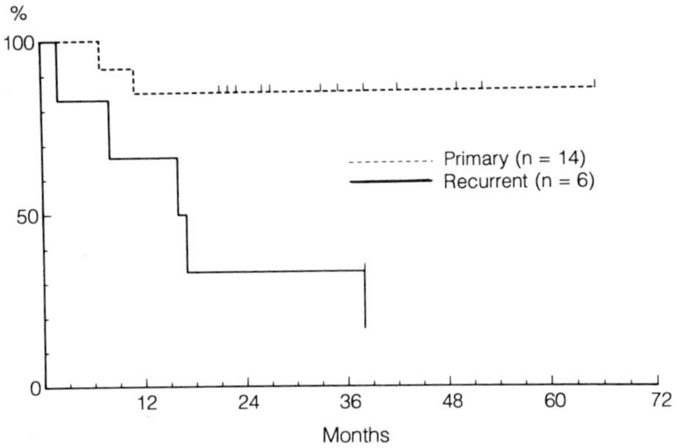

Fig. 14.2. Actuarial survival curves for patients with primary vs recurrent disease at the time of IORT

IORT is an interesting modality that can be included in combined treatment programs. The availability of IORT might decrease the total external beam radiation dose and enable a boost dose to be delivered to areas of residual disease or at high risk for local recurrence, with an accurate and sophisticated electron beam field. The complications observed in our initial series have been due to intensive local treatment. IORT appears to be very attractive for the treatment of Ewing's sarcoma located in central bones (pelvis, vertebra, ribs, etc.), and it is also a feasible technique in lesions of the extremities.

References

Bacci G, Picci P, Gitelis S, Borghi A, Campanacci M (1982) The treatment of localized Ewing's sarcoma. The experience at the Instituo Ortopedico Rizzoli in 163 cases treated with and without adjuvant chemotherapy. Cancer 49: 1561–1570

Brown AP, Fixen JA, Plowman PN (1987) Local control of Ewing's sarcoma: an analysis of 67 patients. Br J Radiol 60: 261–268

Gillette EL, Powers BE, McChesney SL et al. (1988) Response of aorta and branch arteries to experimental intraoperative irradiation. Int J Radiat Oncol Biol Phys 15 [Suppl 1]: 202

Halperin EC, Kun LE, Constine LS, Tarbell NJ (1989) Ewing's sarcoma. In: Halperin EC, Kun LE, Constine LS, Tarbell NJ (eds) Pediatric radiation oncology. Raven New York, pp 187–210

Jurgens H, Exner U, Gadner H et al. (1988) Multidisciplinary treatment of primary Ewing's sarcoma of bone. A 6-year experience of a European Cooperative Trial. Cancer 61: 23–32

Kinsella TJ, Sindelar WF, De Luca AM et al. (1985) Tolerance of peripheral nerve to intraoperative radiotherapy (IORT): clinical and experimental studies. Int J Radiat Oncol Biol Phys 11: 1579–1585

Kinsella TJ, Sindelar WF, De Luca AM (1988) Threshold dose for peripheral nerve injury following intraoperative radiotherapy (IORT) in a large animal model. Int J Radiat Oncol Biol Phys 15 [Suppl 1]: 205

Le Coteur RA, Gillette EL, Powers BE et al. (1989) Peripheral neuropathies following experimental intraoperative radiation therapy (IORT). Int J Radiat Oncol Biol Phys 11: 1579–1585

Malwer MM, Link MP, Donaldson SS (1989) Sarcomas of bone. In: De Vita VT, Hellman S, Rosember SA (eds) Cancer principles and practice of oncology, 3rd edn. JB Lippincott, Philadelphia, pp 1418–1467

Marcus RB, Million RR (1984) The effect of primary tumor size on the prognosis of Ewing's sarcoma. Int J Radiat Oncol Biol Phys 10 [Suppl 1]: 88

Powers BE, Gillette EL, McChesney SL et al. (1989a) Muscle injury following experimental intraopeartive irradiation. Int J Radiat Oncol Biol Phys 17 [Suppl 1]: 246

Powers BE, Gillette EL, McChesney SL et al. (1989b) Bone necrosis and tumor induction following experimental intraoperative irradiation. Int J Radiat Oncol Biol Phys 17: 559–567

Rosen G (1978) Primary Ewing's sarcoma: the multidisciplinary lesion. Int J Radiat Oncol Biol Phys 4: 527–532

Sailder SL, Harmon DC, Mankin HJ, Truman JT, Suit HD (1988) Ewing's sarcoma: surgical resection as a prognostic factor. Int J Radiat Oncol Biol Phys 15: 43–52

Sierrasesúmaga L (1989) Tratamiento multidisciplinario del sarcoma de Ewing. Experiencia en la Clínica Universitaria de Navarra. Doctoral Thesis, University of Navarra, Pamplona (Spain)

Stea B, Kinsella TJ, Triche TJ, Horvath K, Glatstein E, Miser JS (1987) Treatment of pelvic sarcomas in adolescents and young adults with intensive combined modality therapy. Int J Radiat Oncol Biol Phys 13: 1797–1805

Tepper J, Glaubiguer D, Lichter A, Wackenhut J, Glatstein E (1980) Local control of Ewing's sarcoma of bone with radiotherapy and combination chemotherapy. Cancer 46: 1965–1973

15 Osteosarcoma

Felipe A. Calvo, Ignacio Azinovic, Santiago Amillo, José Cañadell, and Luis Sierrasesúmaga

CONTENTS

15.1 Introduction ... 103
15.2 Previous Experiences ... 103
15.2.1 Tissue Tolerance Studies ... 103
15.2.2 Clinical Results ... 104
15.3 Treatment Protocol ... 104
15.4 Analysis of Results ... 105
15.4.1 Patient, Tumor, and Treatment Characteristics ... 105
15.4.2 Toxicity and Complications ... 106
15.4.3 Patterns of Tumor Recurrence and Outcome ... 106
15.5 Conclusion ... 107
References ... 107

15.1 Introduction

The treatment of osteosarcoma has changed dramatically in the last decade. Neoadjuvant and adjuvant chemotherapy has significantly increased both survival and tumor resectability rates (Eilber et al. 1987; Bacci et al. 1987), and extremity preservation is an important goal of modern treatment (Wong et al. 1986). Moreover, while historically osteosarcoma has been considered a "radioresistant" tumor type and there has been a lack of interest in exploring radiotherapy in the multidisciplinary approach to bone tumors (Sugimoto et al. 1989), in recent series this treatment modality has been employed in the local treatment of osteosarcoma of the extremities.

In the era prior to adjuvant chemotherapy the only alternative to amputation for the treatment of the primary lesion was local radiotherapy. The so-called Cade technique was an approach that delivered high dose local irradiation to obtain at least would allow amputation to be delayed for 4–6 months while patients were observed to see whether pulmonary metastases would develop (Jenkin et al. 1972; Allen and Stevens 1973; Poppe et al. 1968; Phillips and Sheline 1969). In the modern practice of radiotherapy, the treatment modality has been reserved for lesions located in sites inaccessible to radical surgery (Chambers and Mahoney 1970; Suit 1975). Several trials have explored the possible role of whole-lung irradiation as an adjuvant treatment for initially localized osteosarcomas (Breur et al. 1978; Burgers et al. 1988). There have also been studies using high dose preoperative irradiation and planned surgery (Farrell and Raventos 1964), and preoperative radiotherapy with local hyperthermic perfusion (Cavaliere 1978).

Intraoperative radiation therapy for the treatment of bone tumors was introduced by a Japanese group (Abe et al. 1988). The treatment program consisted in the use of IORT to treat the involved bone. In the present series IORT was used for the treatment of the tumor bed area and surrounding tissues following bone resection. Moderate to high single doses of electrons were expected to sterilize residual osteosarcoma cells after surgical en bloc tumor resection. In addition, neoadjuvant chemotherapy was employed, since this induces even higher tumor necrosis rates. On the other hand, it was elected to omit external beam radiotherapy in those patients in whom metallic prosthetic devices would have been included in the field. This is the only case in the IORT program in our institution in which IORT was not complemented by external beam irradiation.

Felipe A. Calvo, Dr., Director and Consultant, Ignacio Azinovic, Dr., Radiotherapy Division, Department of Oncology, Santiago Amillo, Dr., José Cañadell, Dr., Consultant, Department of Orthopedic Surgery and Traumatology, Luis Sierrasesúmaga, Dr., Consultant, Pediatric Oncology Unit, Department of Pediatrics, Clinica Universitaria de Navarra, 31080 Pamplona, Spain

15.2 Previous Experiences

15.2.1 Tissue Tolerance Studies

The normal tissues at risk of receiving high to moderate single doses of electron beam in IORT for postresected osteosarcoma of the extremities are muscles, peripheral nerves, ligaments, and skin. Occasionally, structures such as cartilage and bone would be included in the IORT field. These normal tissues have been extensively investigated to define their tolerance to escalating doses of IORT alone or in combination with fractionated external beam radiotherapy (cf. Chap. 13). As mentioned above, in the case of osteosarcoma patients the treatment program in our institution does not include the addition of external beam radiotherapy. The changes in normal tissues described in muscles and peripheral nerves following a 15–20 Gy single dose of IORT alone are compatible with acceptable tolerance, although neurologic damage has been observed in a certain proportion of animals after 20 Gy (Kinsella et al. 1985, 1988; Le Coteur et al. 1989; Powers et al. 1989a,b). This consequently has to be considered the upper dose limit in IORT trials in which nerves will be included in the field.

15.2.2 Clinical Results

The largest clinical experience using IORT in osteosarcoma patients has been reported from Kyoto University (Abe et al. 1989). Between 1978 and 1984 21 patients with osteosarcoma received IORT as a part of the treatment designed for their disease. Involved bones were femur (12), tibia (7), humerus (1), and iliac (1). The primary lesion was treated with IORT alone in 11 cases, while eight patients underwent prosthetic replacement 3 months after IORT. The IORT technique was described as multifocal bilateral irradiation, using electron beams in the energy range of 12–6 MeV and delivering a total dose of 50–60 Gy to an area of the bone determined according to the CT findings. Skin and surrounding tissues were retracted to protect them from the radiation beam. Histologic changes were described in an initial report (Nagashima et al. 1983). Clinical results, published in a later update, showed several findings compatible with treatment efficacy, such as normalization of initially elevated serum alkaline phosphatase, a marked decrease in the uptake of contrast media in bone scintigrams, and complete necrosis of the tumor cells throughout the primary lesions that were resected and analyzed in serial histologic examinations. Two patients developed extensive skin necrosis apparently related to the surgical procedure. The overall cumulative survival was 32%. This has improved since 1982 with the inclusion of chemotherapy in the treatment program; thus the estimated 5-year survival rate in the ten patients treated with the new multidisciplinary program is 60% (Yamamuro et al. 1989). In the most recent update from this group, 2 out of 23 patients are reported to have developed a local recurrence, probably due to a marginal miss of the IORT fields. The most common complication has been fracture of the involved bone. The present recommendation for patients free of distant metastases 8–10 weeks after IORT is reoperation for bone resection and replacement (Abe et al. 1989).

15.3 Treatment Protocol

The treatment protocol has been quite uniform in the patients reviewed in this series. Once osteosarcoma was confirmed histologically, patients were entered in a treatment program comprising three major components:

Neoadjuvant chemotherapy: Three preoperative courses of neoadjuvant chemotherapy were given, commencing at 3-week intervals. Using the transfemoral Seldinger approach, cisplatin 40 mg/m^2 was administered intra-arterially on days 1, 3, and 5 of each cycle. On day 5 of each cycle doxorubicin 60 mg/m^2 i.v. was added to the program.

Surgery: Following the three neoadjuvant courses of chemotherapy, patients were considered for surgical en bloc tumor resection. The general aims of surgery were to remove all the involved bone and a margin of normal surrounding tissues if possible. Functional reconstruction of the extremity was done on an individual basis using endoprosthetic devices or bone graft. Before the reconstruction, the patient received IORT in the tumor bed area, using a single dose in the range of 10–20 Gy. The electron beam energy selected was based on the thickness of tumor tissue left after surgery (Fig. 15.1).

Systemic adjuvant chemotherapy: Three weeks after surgery, intensive adjuvant systemic chemotherapy was initiated using the following regime of cytostatic agents: cisplatin 120 mg/m^2 and doxorubicin 60 mg/m^2 in weeks 1, 5, 15, 25, 33, and 45; high dose methotrexate 8 g/m^2 with folinic acid

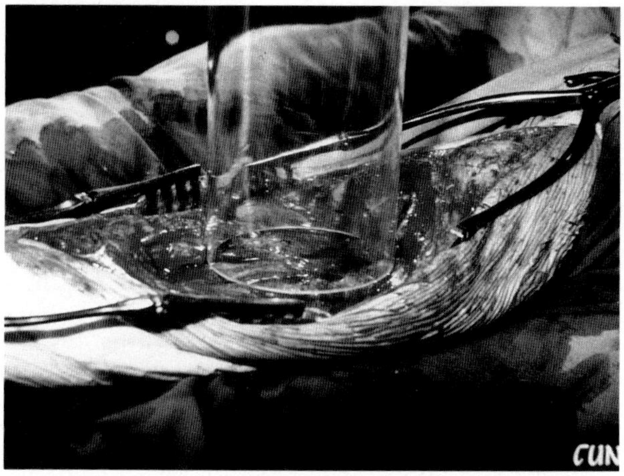

Fig. 15.1. IORT field arrangement for an osteosarcoma of the tibia following resection

rescue in weeks 3, 4, 8, 9, 13, 14, 18, 19, 23, 24, 28, and 29; bleomycin 30 mg/m^2, cyclophosphamide 1200 mg/m^2, vincristine 1.5 mg/m^2, and actinomycin D 1.2 mg/m^2 in weeks 10, 12, 36, 42, and 48.

External beam radiotherapy was not used in this treatment program. Occasionally patients with recurrent and/or macroscopic residual postsurgical disease received additional fractionated irradiation.

Table 15.1. Patient (n = 25) and tumor characteristics in cases of osteosarcoma treated with IORT

	No.	%
Patients		
Sex		
Male	11	44
Female	14	56
Karnofsky performance status		
>70%	21	84
<70%	4	16
Age		
Range: 6–33 years		
Median: 15 years		
Symptoms		
Pain	25	100
Palpable tumor	8	32
Impaired mobility	14	56
Others	3	12
Tumors		
Involved bone		
Femur	17	68
Tibia	5	20
Humerus	3	12
Location		
Proximal	9	36
Medial	1	4
Distal	14	56
Mixed	1	4
Histologic subtype		
Chondroblastic	4	16
Osteoblastic	15	60
Fibroblastic	2	8
Mixed	2	8
Others	2	8

15.4 Analysis of Results

15.4.1 Patient, Tumor and Treatment Characteristics

A total of 25 patients with localized osteosarcoma are available for analysis following the multidisciplinary treatment program including IORT boost to the tumor bed at the time of bone resection. Of these 25 patients, 11 were males and 14, females. Karnofsky performance status was equal or superior to 70% in 21 patients. The patients' ages ranged from 6 to 33 years old, with a median of 15 years. The most frequent symptoms at the time of initial consultation were pain (25 cases), impaired mobility (14), and palpable tumor (8).

The bones in which osteosarcoma developed were the femur in 17 cases, the tibia in five cases, and the humerus in three cases. Pathology reports cited the following subtypes of ostesarcoma: chondroblastic (4), osteoblastic (15), fibroblastic (2), mixed histologies (2), and others (2) (Table 15.1).

The general treatment characteristics have been described above. All patients received the planned chemotherapy. Median duration of chemotherapy was 10.8 months (range 6–15 months). The median time from initial diagnosis to IORT was 91.05 days, with a range of 48–468 days (the latter case being a patient with recurrent disease which was treated again with surgery and IORT plus external beam radiotherapy in an effort to rescue a local failure). An important aspect in the treatment of osteosarcoma is the grade of tumor necrosis observed following neoadjuvant chemotherapy. In our series 14 patients achieved tumor necrosis equal or superior to 90%.

The IORT technique employed consisted in the use of a total of 31 fields. A single field was used in 20 patients, while five required multiple adjacent fields to encompass the target volume adequately. Cone diameter ranged from 5 to 12 cm; in 18 procedures cones of 8, 9, and 10 cm were used, and in ten procedures, a cone of 12 cm. The electron beam energy selected was 6 MeV in 18 cases,

9 MeV in seven, 12 MeV in five, and 15 MeV in one. The total single radiation dose delivered with IORT was 10 Gy in five cases, 15 Gy in 16, and 20 Gy in ten. The major vascular and peripheral nerve structures were included in the IORT beam in 14 cases and were excluded or protected in 11 cases.

External beam radiotherapy was given on an individualized basis in accordance with clinical findings. Five patients received a 5-week course of fractionated external beam radiotherapy of 40–45 Gy for the following reasons: initially marginal resectability in a large tumor not responding to initial chemotherapy (one case; the patient received preoperative radiotherapy); local recurrence following treatment without IORT, and treated again with surgery, IORT boost, and external beam irradiation (one case); chondroblastic osteosarcoma (two cases); and macroscopic residual disease after surgery (one case).

The surgical component of the treatment program included in all cases a wide resection of the bone and surrounding tissues involved by tumor. The repair of the surgical defect was achieved using different prosthetic devices, bone graft, or other surgical techniques. Following bone and soft tissue resection, macroscopic residual tumor was considered to be left in four cases, and microscopic residual disease in 21 cases (Table 15.2).

Table 15.2. Treatment characteristics in cases of osteosarcoma

	No.	%
Surgery		
Macroscopic residual disease	4	16
Microscopic residual disease	21	84
Chemotherapy		
Duration		
Median: 10.8 months		
Range: 6–15 months		
Tumor necrosis		
<90%	11	44
>90%	14	56
Radiotherapy		
IORT[a]		
Number of fields		
Single	20	80
Multiple	5	20
Cone diameter (cm)		
5–7	3	10
8–10	18	58
12	10	22
Total dose (Gy)		
10	5	16
15	16	52
20	10	32
Electron energy (MeV)		
6	18	58
9	7	22
12	5	16
15	1	4
External beam		
Preoperative	1	4
Postoperative	4	16

[a] Total number of fields treated = 31

15.4.2 Toxicity and Complications

A wide variety of toxic events and complications were observed in this series of patients as a result of the intensive systemic and locoregional treatment program. For the purpose of the present analysis, only those observations that might be related to IORT in one way or another were included. In the long-term follow-up of patients a certain degree of functional limitation of the treated extremity was observed in 16 patients. Six had evident dysmetria. In seven patients atrophy was present. Three patients developed clinically symptomatic peripheral neuropathy with motor and sensory deficits and were documented with electrophysiologic studies. One of these patients recovered partially from the symptoms. All patients who developed neuropathy were treated with 20 Gy IORT. Three of the patients treated with a combination of IORT and external beam radiotherapy developed both extremity atrophy and dysmetria.

Local infections were seen postoperatively in four patients, requiring removal of the implanted device in two cases.

One patient had a recall phenomenon in the IORT field each time high dose methotrexate was administered during adjuvant chemotherapy. It consisted in the development of transient skin erythema describing the IORT exit beam in the posterior portion of the leg.

15.4.3 Patterns of Tumor Recurrence and Outcome

The median follow-up time for the entire series at the time of this analysis was 19 months, with a range of 1–52+ months. There has been one combined failure (local and systemic) at 9 months after IORT treatment in a patient with macroscopic residual disease and less than 90% tumor necrosis.

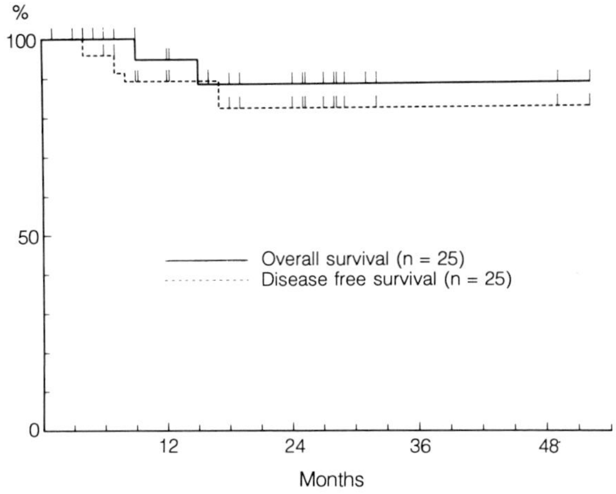

Fig. 15.2. Actuarial disease-free and overall survival curves in osteosarcoma patients

The initial sites of metastasis were the lungs (4), pleura (1), peritoneum (1), bone (1), and soft tissues (1), in the three patients who have shown disease progression.

At the present time 23 patients are alive and two have died. Actuarial survival is 87% and disease-free survival, 83% (Fig. 15.2).

15.5 Conclusion

The significant changes that have taken place in the management of patients with osteosarcoma in recent years, with the successful use of both neoadjuvant and adjuvant chemotherapy, have increased interest in the local treatment of osteosarcoma of the extremities. Limb-sparing procedures have been employed widely and constitute one of the most challenging areas of research in contemporary surgical oncology. Radiation therapy is not considered a useful treatment modality in osteosarcoma patients. This is surprising if one considers that the combination of surgery and radiotherapy has become the standard recommended treatment for soft tissue sarcomas of the extremities (Rosenberg et al. 1982). The difference in radiation resistance between these histologic tumor subtypes is not so extreme and is reduced even further if the amount of postsurgical residual disease is minimal.

The goal of osteosarcoma treatment today is not only systemic disease control but also extremity preservation, and in this context the addition of IORT might improve local control rates. External beam radiotherapy might be more hazardous in osteosarcoma patients who have undergone resection owing to the interaction of the radiation with metallic prosthetic reconstructive devices and the intensive chemotherapy programs required to cure these patients. As with soft tissue sarcomas, the tolerance of peripheral nerves to single high doses of electrons is an important and still open question.

References

Abe M, Takahashi M, Shibamoto Y, Ono K, Yabumoto E, Mori, K (1988) Derzeitige Stellung der intraoperativen Strahlentherapie. Chirurg 59: 211–217

Abe M, Takahashi M, Shibamoto Y, Ono K (1989) Application of intraoperative radiation therapy to refractory cancers. Ann Radiol 32: 493–494

Allen CF, Stevens KR (1973) Preoperative irradiation for osteogenic sarcoma. Cancer 31: 1364–1366

Bacci G, Springfield D, Capnna R et al. (1987) Neoadjuvant chemotherapy for osteosarcoma of the extremity. Clin Orthop 224: 268–276

Breur K, Cohen P, Schweisguth O, Hart Amm (1978) Irradiation of the lungs or an adjuvant therapy in the treatment of osteosarcoma of the limbs. An EORTC randomized study. Eur J Cancer 14: 461–471

Burgers JM, van Glabbeke M, Bussan A et al. (1988) Osteosarcoma of the limbs. Report of the EORTC-SIOP 03 trial 20781 investigating the value of adjuvant treatment with chemotherapy and/or prophylactic lung irradiation. Cancer 61: 1024–1031

Cavaliere R (1978) Hyperthermic treatment of osteogenic sarcoma. Chemother Oncol 2: 190–196

Chambers RG, Mahoney WD (1970) Osteogenic sarcoma of the mandible: current management. Am Surg 36: 463–471

Eilber F, Giuliano A, Edkardt J, Patterson K, Moselev S, Goodnight J (1987) Adjuvant chemotherapy for osteosarcoma: a randomized prospective trial. J Clin Oncol 5: 21–26

Farrell C, Raventos A (1964) Experiences in treating osteosarcoma at the hospital of the University of Pennsylvania. Radiology 83: 1080–1083

Jenkin RDT, Allt WEC, Fitzpatrick PJ (1972) Osteosarcoma: an assessment of management with particular reference to primary irradiation and selective delayed amputation. Cancer 30: 393–400

Kinsella TJ, Sindelar WF, de Luca AM et al. (1985) Tolerance of peripheral nerve to intraoperative radiotherapy (IORT): clinical and experimental studies. Int J Radiat Oncol Biol Phys 11: 1579–1585

Kinsella TJ, Sindelar WF, de Luca AM (1988) Threshold dose for peripheral nerve injury following intraoperative radiotherapy (IORT) in a large animal model. Int J Radiat Oncol Biol Phys 15 [Suppl 1]: 205

Le Coteur RA, Gillette EL, Powers BE et al. (1989) Peripheral neuropathies following experimental intraoperative radiation therapy (IORT). Int J Radiat Oncol Biol Phys 17: 583–590

Nagashima T, Yamamuro T, Kotoura Y, Takahashi M, Abe M (1983) Histological studies of the effect of intraoperative irradiation on osteosarcoma. Nippon Seikeigeka Gakkai Zasshi 57: 1681–1697

Phillips TL, Sheline GE (1969) Radiation therapy of malignant bone tumors. Radiology 92: 1537–1545
Poppe E, Liverud K, Efskind J (1968) Osteosarcoma. Acta Chir Scand 134: 549–556
Powers BE, Gillette EL, McChesney SL et al. (1989a) Muscle injury following experimental intraoperative irradiation. Int J Radiat Oncol Biol Phys 17 [Suppl 1]: 246
Powers BE, Gillette EL, McChesney SL et al. (1989b) Bone necrosis and tumor induction following experimental intraoperative irradiation. Int J Radiat Oncol Biol Phys 17: 559–567
Rosenberg SA, Tepper JE, Glatstein EJ et al. (1982) The treatment of soft tissue sarcomas of the extremities. Prospective randomized evaluations of (1) limb-sparing surgery plus radiation therapy compared with amputation and (2) the role of adjuvant chemotherapy. Ann Surg 196: 305–314
Sugimoto M, Togochida J, Kotoura Y, Yamamuro T, Utsumi H (1989) In vitro radiosensitivity of osteosarcoma lines. Strahlenther Onkol 165: 782
Suit HD (1975) Radiotherapy in osteosarcoma. Clin Orthop 111: 71–75
Wong ACW, Akahoshi Y, Takeuchi S (1986) Limb-salvage procedures for osteosarcoma: an alternative to amputation. Int Orthop 10: 245–251
Yamamuro T, Kotoura Y, Kasahara K, Tadahashi M, Abe M (1989) Intraoperative radiotherapy for osteosarcoma. Strahlenther Onkol 165: 783

16 Summary and Future Prospects

Felipe A. Calvo, Manuel Santos, and Luther W. Brady

CONTENTS

16.1 Indications in Tumors of Multiple Sites 109
16.1.1 Feasibility 109
16.1.2 Definition of the Target Volume 110
16.2 Clinical Tolerance of Intensive Locoregional Treatment Programs 110
16.2.1 IORT plus External Beam Radiotherapy 110
16.2.2 IORT-Sensitive Tissues and Structures 111
16.3 Summary of Clinical Results 112
16.3.1 Local Tumor Control 112
16.3.2 Survival Data 113
16.4 Future Prospects 114
References 114

16.1 Indications in Tumors of Multiple Sites

The role of IORT as a sophisticated electron boosting modality for unresectable tumors or areas at high risk for local recurrence following resection has to be studied in a variety of sites. The use of IORT during cancer surgery in different anatomic locations will help to develop the technical skills required to implement a safe and active program. This combined approach will, at the same time, yield enough significant information for an assessment to be made as to which tumor sites can be regarded as suitable for the testing of IORT in large prospective clinical studies (Rich 1986; Kinsella et al. 1988).

Felipe A. Calvo, Dr., Director and Consultant, Manuel Santos, Dr., Radiotherapy Division, Department of Oncology, Clinica Universitaria de Navarra, 31080 Pamplona, Spain

Luther W. Brady, MD, Professor and Chairman, Hahnemann University, Department of Radiation Oncology and Nuclear Medicine, Broad & Vine, Mail Stop 200, Philadelphia, PA 19102–1192, USA

16.1.1 Feasibility

Use of IORT during cancer surgery is feasible in most tumor locations. We did not find difficulties in patient transportation to be a contraindication to IORT. The most difficult transportation position was the lithotomy position; in general, these were patients treated for presacral recurrences through a transperineal approach. IORT has not been limited by factors related to anesthetic support. Patients who underwent prolonged surgical procedures and/or required large quantities of blood were stabilized before transportation. These patients had in most cases undergone complicated pelvic surgery, such as exenterations or other surgical approaches for recurrent disease. Special care was needed in patients who underwent thoracic surgery (in general with the diagnosis of lung cancer), some of whom had cardiopulmonary compromise. Patients with intracranial, head and neck, upper abdominal, and extremity tumors were in general treated with IORT without major difficulties.

Another interesting feature is the technical limitations on the use of IORT in some anatomic areas. In our experience, tumors involving the anterior part of the chest wall or abdominal wall were not amenable to IORT due to technical limitations in positioning the IORT cone. An example of this type of difficulty was a case of mesothelioma in which portions of the parietal pleura could not be treated. Another situation in which IORT might be contraindicated is when large tumors are located in anatomic cavities in which the IORT cone will not adequately cover the postsurgical target volume. A final possible contraindication is situations where the amount of normal tissues that will have to be included in the IORT field will be so great as to negate the benefits of IORT, and where the patient would benefit more from the use of more conventional treatment; an example is large unresectable tumors in the upper abdomen with fixation of the tumor to small bowel, colon, etc.

16.1.2 Definition of the Target Volume

An issue of particular importance in the design of IORT protocols, and the evaluation of the results, is the definition of the target volume for IORT. In most cases in which this modality is used for the treatment of unresectable tumors or partially resected masses, the target volume will be clearly defined as the area of residual disease plus a margin of normal tissues. This can be assessed by means of tumor palpation, direct visualization of the surgical area, and/or more sophisticated diagnostic techniques such as intraoperative ultrasound (SCHOENECKER et al. 1986). It is particularly important to measure accurately the thickness of the tumor or residual disease. Pancreatic cancer is a typical example of this situation. There are, however, some special indications for IORT in which it is employed in an adjuvant fashion to treat locoregional nodal drainage areas. The definition of the target tumor volume is more complicated in these cases. In our experience examples of this type of indication are gastric cancer and lung cancer, in which the upper abdominal and mediastinal nodal areas, respectively, were treated following resection of the primary lesion. In these cases IORT does not encompass known tumor, but an anatomic region at risk of microscopic residual disease. The target volume has to be carefully defined at the time of surgery. The data gathered will determine the size of the IORT cones employed or, more strictly, the IORT area to be treated (which varies with the cone diameter and the angle of beveled cone used). An intermediate situation between these two extremes (measurable disease after surgery and adjuvant treatment) is represented by tumors that have been removed with surgical margins. Such cases are reported as involving treatment of "the tumor bed or areas at high risk for local recurrence". Examples of such indications are head and neck cancer and soft tissue or bone sarcomas. Again, it has to be decided whether the IORT treatment area will be limited to the inclusion of surgical margins, or whether the aim of the treatment will be to cover all the surgically manipulated tissue by the use of larger field sizes.

In many instances the definition of the target volume will entail the question of whether a single or multiple field technique should be employed to encompass the selected treatment area (SHAW et al. 1987). We are now very much in favor of using single fields. The reproducibility of IORT clinical data depends largely on this small but important point. Other relevant aspects of the technique such as the type of surgical intervention, the electron energy, the total IORT dose, and the cone size are parameters that will not vary significantly from institution to institution. In contrast the normal tissue toxicity and local tumor control data might be altered by the use of multiple field techniques, which will imply larger target volumes and/or areas of overlapping fields. Thus in our opinion use of the multiple field technique should be limited to those occasional cases that require an extra small volume to treat the target area. In summary, with the reproducibility of clinical data in mind, we recommend IORT protocol designs in which single fields are employed and multiple fields used only when absolutely necessary.

16.2 Clinical Tolerance of Intensive Locoregional Treatment Programs

The clinical tolerance to intensive cancer therapy is a critical issue for the future of any treatment modality (BRADY et al. 1990). As a rule it appears in clinical oncology that the initial testing of treatment intensification programs will give rise to associated toxicities and complications, but that when the experiences are consolidated and the indications and techniques refined, most of these problems will be overcome. In the case of IORT integrated in multidisciplinary treatment programs, the clinical tolerance is related to the combination of extensive radical surgery, systemic chemotherapy, and high dose radiotherapy. Since IORT is a developing modality, many patients considered candidates for the modality have had recurrences following previous treatments or locally advanced tumor stages. Therefore, another important factor which should be considered when evaluating tolerance to a treatment program is a compromised performance status at the initiation of treatment. All these factors together have to be at least mentioned at the time of publishing reports on IORT, particularly the data related to toxicity and complications observed.

16.2.1 IORT plus External Beam Radiotherapy

Our review has made available a significant amount of information from which conclusions can be drawn on the locoregional tolerance of normal tissues, organs, and structures to IORT plus external beam radiotherapy. In general the tolerance of normal tissues to moderate doses of IORT (10–15 Gy) plus a full course of external beam radiotherapy has been acceptable. It is important to note that in those protocols in which this type of approach was used, the tolerance was reasonably good but there were noticeable clinical changes. It has to be mentioned at this point that some cases of esophagitis, pneumonitis, and long-term lung fibrosis occurred using the treatment program developed for lung cancer patients, and that soft tissue fibrosis was observed in some patients with sarcoma of the extremities. With the gastric cancer protocol only a few complications resulted from the combination of external beam radiotherapy and IORT boost to the celiac axis; examples include vertabral collapse, development of liver hemangiomas in patients with long-term fibrosis in the vessels of the celiac trunk, and reversible cases of elevated liver enzyme levels (probably related to the inclusion of the left hepatic lobe in the field of the external beam).

An exceptional situation in our series is represented by a few patients with Ewing's sarcoma who developed soft tissue necrosis in the area of high dose radiotherapy and surgical manipulation. As was explained in the corresponding chapter, these patients belonged to a small group of patients with large primary tumor masses in which the treatment program was modified and preoperative flash irradiation (10 Gy) was administered 24–48 h before surgery. In these patients the rest of the radiotherapy program was given to full course; under such circumstances the final radiation dose reached in the target volume will produce major tissue changes, even without surgical manipulation.

Analysis of the data obtained with the different IORT protocols tested in our institution shows that although the tolerance is acceptable, the treatment programs are close to the maximum limit of a relatively safe combination of surgery, fractionated external beam irradiation, and IORT boost.

16.2.2 IORT-Sensitive Tissues and Structures

The review of the clinical reports on the use of IORT has identified three structures as showing a degree of tissue damage from IORT greater than would have been predicted theoretically: the duodenum (Sindelar et al. 1985), the ureters, and the peripheral nerves (Shaw et al. 1990). Animal experiments have been consistent with the clinical observations (Le Coteur et al. 1989; Ahmadu-Suka et al. 1988).

In our own series some of the initial unexpected toxicities were related to the tolerance of some of the aforementioned tissues to a high single dose of electrons followed by external beam radiotherapy. For example, we observed neuropathy in several patients with pelvic tumors or sarcomas of the extremities. After such observations were made the IORT does was decreased in an effort to avoid these complications. Further analysis will reveal whether this decision will affect the rates of complications and/or local tumor control.

We observed distinctive alterations of the ureters if they were included in the IORT field, but the data are rather unclear because (a) many patients treated with pelvic tumors underwent pelvic exenteration and (b) pelvic surgery was performed by a number of different surgical teams.

Late duodenitis and gastrointestinal bleeding were also seen, although the incidence of these complications was low. In the case of pancreatic cancer, the patients who developed these complications most frequently were those with metastases who were treated by IORT for abdominal pain. These patients in general had large primary tumors, so that the duodenum had to be included in the IORT field; most had liver metastases, and in addition there were alterations in the coagulation system and very poor performance status. The combination of these factors made in difficult to evaluate the importance of each component in the development of the complication.

Several isolated observations might have been related to IORT tissue toxicity, but the number of cases was too small for a definite conclusion to be drawn. Such observations were made with different treatment protocols. The most prominent were an acute episode of brain edema, a case of long-term myelopathy (in a patient with posterior neck sarcoma), and a left gastric artery stump which developed an aneurysm and eventual rupture.

The bronchial stump was considered to be a sensitive structure in an early clinical series at the National Cancer Institute (USA) (Pass et al. 1987). This has not been confirmed in our own review. The thoracic surgeons in our institution contributed the idea of using vascularized pleural or pericardial flaps to cover the bronchial suture following the delivery of IORT in that area. This is an example of surgical input in the development of IORT programs.

16.3 Summary of Clinical Results

The clinical experience obtained in our institution is reported in this monograph, grouping the patients by tumor site and/or histologic type and following the style of previous authors on the subject to facilitate the interpretation of the data. As the reader may have noted, the number of patients treated in the period 1984–1989 and recorded in Tables 1.1 and 1.2 are at variance with the actual number of patients analyzed in each chapter according to tumor site. These differences have arisen for three major reasons: first, a minority of patients were not eligible for analysis due to the presence of metastatic disease at the time of IORT; second, patients with miscellaneous histologies or tumor sites treated with IORT were not included; third, in some instances the period of time analyzed did not extend to December 1989, which was the time limit for Tables 1.1 and 1.2.

16.3.1 Local Tumor Control

Promotion of local tumor control is the ultimate aim of integration of IORT in multidisciplinary oncology. An overview of the results obtained in this series seems an important final task.

When studying local control, several factors have to be taken into account in assessing the value of IORT. These factors include the tumor burden left after surgery, the site of treatment, and the status of the disease treated (primary vs recurrent tumors). In our analysis, local failure included any tumor recurrence in the locoregional structures included in or marginal to the IORT field (the latter cases indicate poor IORT technique) but definitely included in the external beam field.

The tumor sites considered for local control evaluation were those in which IORT has been employed in a significant number of patients, with achievement of median follow-up time.

16.3.1.1 Postsurgical Residual Disease

Table 16.1 summarizes the results regarding the relationship between postsurgical residual disease and the number of local failures in several tumor sites. The limitations of such an analysis are evident, but it might serve as a point of departure in illustrating that local tumor control in different tumor sites might be related to the actual tumor burden treated by IORT, with or without surgery and external beam radiotherapy. Patients with bladder cancer and intracranial tumors are excluded from this analysis.

Table 16.1. Local control, tumor sites/tumor, and postsurgical residual disease in patients treated with IORT

Tumor site/tumor	Postsurgical residual disease		No resection LF/#
	Microscopic LF/#	Macroscopic LF/#	
Head and neck	5/11	5/6	0/0
Lung	1/13	2/29	9/18
Gastric	4/32	4/6	1/2
Pancreas	0/0	0/0	7/25
Colorectal	0/36	7/8	3/5
Gynecologic	1/7	6/16	3/4
Ewing's sarcoma	0/13	1/4	0/3
STS, extremities	1/17	1/2	0/0
STS, central	4/11	6/12	1/1
Osteosarcoma	0/22	1/3	0/0
Local control rates	90%	62%	59%

Abbreviations: #, total number of patients in the group; LF, number of local failures; STS, soft tissue sarcomas

16.3.1.2 Tumor Location

A question that has rarely been addressed in IORT trials is whether the tumor location is a factor of relevance for the final results or whether IORT can treat with similar success any anatomic site in the human body. Table 16.2 reviews the results obtained in our series. It is interesting to

Table 16.2. Local control and tumor location in patients treated with IORT

Tumor location	No. of patients	Local failures	Local control
Head and neck	21	12	43%
Intrathoracic	67	14	79%
Upper abdomen	71	20	72%
Pelvis	87	24	72%
Extremities	60	3	95%

Table 16.3. Local control and disease status: comparison of results in recurrent vs locally advanced primary tumors (abbreviations as in Table 16.1)

Tumor site/tumor	Disease status	
	Recurrent LF/#	Primary LF/#
Head and neck	9/13	1/4
Lung	0/0	12/60
Gastric	1/2	8/38
Pancreas	0/0	7/25
Colorectal	10/28	0/21
Gynecology	5/15	5/12
Ewing's sarcoma	0/6	1/14
STS, extremities	1/12	1/7
STS, central	7/12	4/12
Osteosarcoma	0/0	1/25
Local control rates	63%	82%

note that the extremities are very easily treated with IORT, that high local control rates might be expected in rather "resistant" histologic tumor subtypes, and that the pelvis is the technically most difficult anatomic area, which might have a significant effect on the outcome that can be achieved in this region.

16.3.1.3 Disease Status: Recurrent Versus Primary Tumors

An analysis performed in many IORT reports is a comparison of survival in patients with recurrent disease and patients with locally advanced primary tumors. Recurrences of most human tumors carry a higher risk of systemic dissemination of disease and necessitate a more complicated and limited surgical approach. The interrelation of these factors in the final results of IORT treatment protocols can only be analyzed in studies involving a large series of patients. Our series has many limitations due to heterogeneity in several treatment and disease parameters, but it does provide information confirming that recurrent disease is a poor prognostic feature. When possible, data in respect of recurrent and primary disease should be reported and analyzed separately (Table 16.3).

16.3.2 Survival Data

Figures 16.1–16.3 show the actuarial survival curves for the different tumor sites treated and analyzed. No separate analysis has been per-

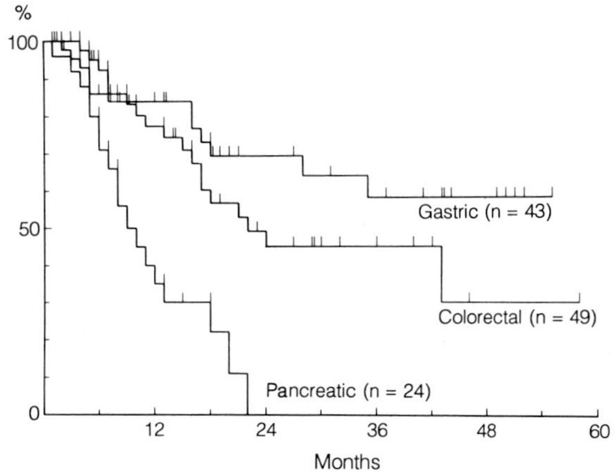

Fig. 16.1. Actuarial survival curves for the groups of patients with gastrointestinal cancer treated with IORT

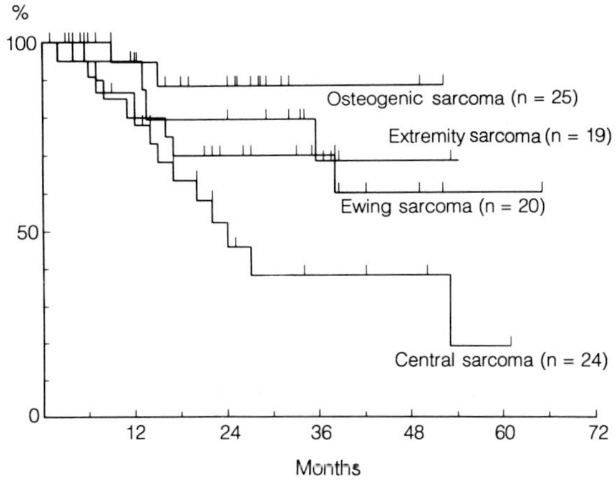

Fig. 16.2 Actuarial survival curves for patients with soft tissue and bone sarcomas treated with IORT

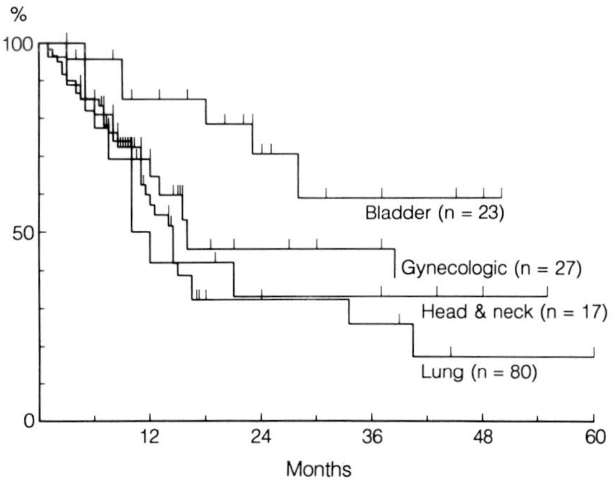

Fig. 16.3 Actuarial survival curves for patients with bladder, gynecologic, head and neck, and lung cancer treated with IORT

formed for subsets of patients based on prognostic factors. The survival data give an overview of what can be achieved at the present time in multidisciplinary oncology when a sophisticated electron boost is delivered at the time of cancer surgery. The selection of tumor sites for IORT trials has to be based upon the local control rates that can be obtained with locoregional intensification treatment programs, but the final survival data will be influenced by tumor behavior and particularly the tendency toward early distant dissemination.

16.4 Future Prospects

Over the past decade IORT has proven to be a feasible, safe, and well tolerated treatment modality for patients undergoing cancer surgery. The local tumor control rates reported by many groups suggest improved tumor control compared with standard treatment modalities.

The work initiated in the 1980s needs to be continued during the present decade. Various clinical and technical aspects need to be addressed. IORT will have to be introduced in more institutions and requires wider acceptance by our surgical colleagues (Wolkov et al. 1988). The final test for this local treatment modality would be in the frame of phase III trials.

References

Ahmadu-Suka F, Gillette EL, Withrow SJ, Husted PW, Nelson AW, Whiteman C (1988) Pathologic response of the pancreas and duodenum to experimental intraoperative radiation. Int J Radiat Oncol Biol Phys 14: 1197–1204

Brady LW, Markoe AM, Micaily B, Fisher SA, Lamm FR (1990) Innovative techniques in radiation oncology. Clinical research programs to improve local and regional control in cancer. Cancer 65: 610–624

Kinsella TJ, Sindelar WF, Tepper JE, Tochner Z, Rich TA (1988) Intraoperative radiotherapy. In: Withers HR, Peters LJ (eds) Innovations in radiation oncology. Springer, Berlin Heidelberg New York, pp 143–153

Le Coteur RA, Gillette EL, Powers BE et al. (1989) Peripheral neuropathies following experimental intraoperative radiation therapy (IORT). Int J Radiat Oncol Biol Phys 11: 1579–1585

Pass HI, Sindelar WF, Kinsella TJ et al. (1987) Delivery of intraoperative radiation therapy after pneumonectomy: experimental observations and early clinical results. Ann Thorac Surg 44: 14–20

Rich TA (1986) Intraoperative radiotherapy. Radiother Oncol 6: 207–221

Schoenecker SA, Mack LA, Russell AH, Cyr DR, Shuman WP, Lennard ES, Montana MA (1986) Intraoperative US as an aid to intraoperative electron beam radiation therapy. Radiology 160: 251–253

Shaw EG, Blackwell CR, McCullough EC, Gunderson LL (1987) Resident essay award: matching intraoperative electron-beam fields: dosimetric and clinical considerations. Int J Radiat Oncol Biol Phys 13: 1303–1307

Shaw EG, Gunderson LL, Martin JK et al. (1990) Peripheral nerve and ureteral tolerance of intraoperative radiation therapy: clinical and dose-response analysis. Radiother Oncol 18: 247–255

Sindelar WF, Kinsella TJ, Hoekstra HJ, Tocher ZA, Smith R, Maher MM (1985) Duodenal hemorrhage as a complication of intraoperative radiotherapy for unresectable carcinomas of the pancreas (abstract C-1075). Proc Am Soc Clin Oncol 4: 277

Wolkov HB, Chenery SG, Asche DR et al. (1988) Practical and technical considerations in establishing an intraoperative radiation therapy program in a community practice. Radiology 168: 255–258

Subject Index

abcess
– pelvic 66, 80, 82
– pulmonary 54
accelerator (see linear accelerator)
alkaline phosphatase 104
amputation 95, 101
– osteosarcoma 103
– salvage treatment 95, 96
amylase 52
anesthesia 25
– drugs 27
– maintenance 29
– neuroleptoanesthesia 26
– ventilation 28, 30
aneurysm 54, 111
applicator 11, 17–22
arrythmias, risk of 2, 5
astrocytoma 31, 32, 35
– anaplastic 33
– glioblastoma multiforme 33
– mixed histology 33
atrophy 106
autopsy 48, 58
– Ewing's
– lung 48
– pancreas 58

base of the tongue, carcinoma 38
beam
– central ray 11, 14
– entrance point 11
– flatness 15, 16, 19
– horns 15, 21, 22
– penumbra 15, 17, 19, 21, 22
– profiles 14–17, 19, 21, 22
– symetry 15, 16, 19
bile duct stricture 52, 58, 61
bilio-digestive bypass 57
bleeding
– arterial 80
– esophageal 54
– gastrointestinal 52, 54, 58, 61, 87, 111
– – arterial fistula 66
– – duodenitis 58, 61, 111
– pelvic 82
– rectal
– – perineal 70
bolus 21, 31, 33
bone fracture 104
bone graft 106
brachial plexus 48, 49
brachytherapy 37, 43, 85
– bladder 73
brain edema 32, 33, 34, 35
– fatal complication 32
brain metastasis 32
brain tumors (see chapter 4)
Bremsstrahlung 13, 14, 19, 22
bronchial stump 44, 45, 50
– dehiscence 45
bronchopleural fistula 45, 48
build-up 93 (see bolus)

calcifications 76
calibration 11, 19
cardiomyopathy 96
carinal necrosis 45
carotid artery 37, 38
– rupture 38
CEA 68
chemoimmunotherapy 65
chemotherapy 3, 4, 25, 31
– ACNU 32
– actinimycin D 105
– bleomycin 105
– carboplatin 67
– cisplatin 33, 54, 60, 75, 81, 94, 104
– cyclophosphamide 105
– dacarbacine 94
– doxorubicin 75, 94, 104
– 5-fluorouracil 54, 59, 60, 67, 75, 81
– gastric 54
– hexamethylmelamine 75
– ifosfamide 94
– methotrexate 104
– nitroureas 31
– pancreas 59, 60
– rectal 67
– vincristine 105
chest wall instability 48, 49
cholangitis 54, 61
clinical trials (see studies)
coagulative necrosis 44
collimators 15, 17
coma 33
complications
– accidental endotracheal extubation 30
– diffuse hemorrhage 30
– massive hemorrhage, clip release 30
Coulomb's law 13
craniotomy 31
cystitis 68
cystometry 74

delayed wound healing 66, 70, 101
depth-dose 11–14, 19, 21
diarrhea 54, 61
distance, correction factors 19, 20
dose
– absorbed 12, 14, 16, 21
– depth of 13, 20–22
– distribution 14, 16, 18, 19
– maximum 13
– peripheral 15, 17, 19, 22
– rate 20
– surface 19, 21
dosimetry 19
dumping 54, 61
dysmetria 106
dysphagia 54

edema 76
– brain 111
– leg 80, 82
electric fields 13
electron
– range 13, 14
– secondary 12–14
electrophysiologic studies 68, 91
endarteritis 44
enteritis 87
ependymoma 34
equilibrium
– electronic 12, 13
– lateral 15
esophageal 44, 45
– fistula 45
– stenosis 45
– ulceration 44, 45
esophagitis 45, 48, 49, 111
external beam radiotherapy 5, 25, 26

femoral fracture 95
fibrosis
– adventitial 44
– bladder 74
– – extensive 76
– – submucosal 74
– – teleangiectasia 74
– Ewing's 101
– lung 48, 49, 89
– porta hepatis 58
– soft tissue 95, 96, 111
– subintimal (artery) 58
fistula
– perineal 68
– vesicovaginal 82

gastrectomy 52
gastric cancer, stump recurrence 54

head and neck cancer (see chapter 5)
– basal cell, recurrent 38
– melanoma 38
– salivary gland 38
– sarcoma 38
– squamous cell carcinoma 38

hemangiosarcoma 74
hemipelvectomy 87
hemoptysis 48, 49
hemostasis 2, 3, 28, 29, 30
hydronephrosis, bilateral 74
hyperthermia 3, 59
– perfusion (osteosarcoma) 103
hypotension, risk of 2, 5
hypoxic cells 2
– sensitizers 4, 59
– – misonidazole 59

ileitis 68
ileus, prolonged 80, 82
iliac vein thrombosis 82
infection, postoperative 30
insulin 52
internal jugular vein 37, 38
inverse square law 20, 21
ionization 14
isodose
– charts 17
– curves 16–17, 19
– surfaces 16, 17

jaundice 60

linear accelerators 16
liver
– biliary cirrhosis 58
– cholestasis 58
– enzymes 111
– hemangioma 52, 54, 111
– infarction 54
– necrosis 58
– steatosis 58
lobectomy 45, 47
lung
– fibrosis 111
– non small cell 43
– small cell 43, 46
lymphocele 82

mediastinal 44, 45, 49
– nodal sampling 45
– recurrence 49
– tolerance 44
melanoma, metastatic posterior fossa 32
meningioma 32, 33, 34, 35
mesothelioma 109
multi-institutional 35
– trials 3
myelopathy 89, 111
myocutaneous flaps 3, 37, 38, 39
– repair 101

necrosis
– skin 104
– soft tissue 101, 111
neoadjuvant chemotherapy
– bladder 73, 76, 77
– lung 43, 46, 47
– osteosarcoma 103, 107
– sarcoma 94
nerve degeneration, pancreas 58
neuroblastoma, intracraneal 34
neuropathy 87, 89, 91, 95, 106
– pain 80, 82, 95
– pelvic
– – pain 66, 67, 68, 70
– – numbness 66
– – weakness 66
– weakness 82
normal tissue toxicity 2
– blood vessels 2
– lung 2
– peripheral nerves 2
– small bowel 2
– ureter 2
nutritional deficiency 58

oligodendroglioma 33, 34
osteoradionecrosis 38
output factors 19

pain
– abdominal 7
– palliation 57, 62
– pelvic 5
Pancoast 46, 47, 48
pancreatic
– fibrosis 51, 58
– – atrophy 51, 58
– – atypical epithelial changes in the ducts 58
– – exocrine insufficiency 51, 58
– fistula 52
paresthesia 48, 49
peripheral nerve, tolerance 32
phantom 14, 17
pleural effusion 54
pneumonectomy 45, 47
pneumonitis 44, 48, 49, 86, 89, 111
posterior fossa 32
preoperative radiotherapy 5
– bladder 73
– Ewing's 100
– lung 43, 47
– osteosarcoma 103, 106
– pancreas 62
– rectal 65, 66
– sarcoma 86
previous irradiation, recurrence to 3
prosthesis 103, 104, 106, 107
protocol design 3
pulmonary artery rupture 48, 49

quality control 3, 4, 5
quality of life 7
quality of therapy 7

radiation
– beams 11, 13
– characteristic 14
– electromagnetic 14
– secondary 13
radiation sensitizers 3
(see hypoxic cell)
radiobiology 2
randomized studies 71, 87, 90, 91
recall phenomenon 106
rejected foreign body 76
rib fracture 48, 49
rupture, superior mesenteric artery 58

sarcoma 74
sciatic nerve 82
seizures 33
shielding 46, 92, 96
side-effects, on the skin 12
sigmoid 67
small bowel obstruction 66
spinal cord 53
stenosis, ureterovesical junction 74
sterilization 18
steroids 34, 48
studies
– phase I–II 4, 7
– phase III 4, 8, 35
(see ramdomized studies)
suboclusive intestinal crisis 61, 68, 70
supratentorial, hemispheric 32, 33
surgery 2, 25
suture dehiscence 54, 79, 82

therapeutic index 1, 2
thoracotomy 96
tracheoesophageal fistula 48, 49
transportation, patient 27, 109
– accessory material 28
– lithotomy 109
– sterile conditions 28
treatment planning 11
tumor response, assessment 5
– fibrosis 5
– hematoma 5
– neuropathy 5
– pelvic pain 5
– presacral mass 5

ulcer
– duodenal 58
– gastric 52, 58
ultrasound, intraoperative 110
ureteral obstruction 66, 70, 80, 82, 86, 87
urinary diversion 74
urinary incontinence 82

vagus nerve, tolerance 38
vascular bypass 96
vascular fibrosis 86
vascular sclerosis 58
vascularized flap 44, 45, 47, 50
– pericardial 44, 50
– pleural 44, 50, 111
vena cava laceration 80
venous thrombosis 95
vertebral
– collapse 52, 54, 89, 111
– marrow hypocelluarity 58

x-rays
– contamination 13, 19
– diagnostic 13
– orthovoltage 11

List of Contributors

Dr. Oscar Abuchaibe
Radiotherapy Division
Department of Oncology
Clinica Universitaria de Navarra
E-31080 Pamplona
Spain

Dr. Francisco Aguilera
Director
Neurosurgery Division
Clinica Universitaria de Navarra
E-31080 Pamplona
Spain

Dr. Javier Alvarez-Cienfuegos
Consultant
Department of Surgery
Clinica Universitaria de Navarra
E-31080 Pamplona
Spain

Dr. Santiago Amillo
Department of Orthopedic Surgery
and Traumatology
Clinica Universitaria de Navarra
E-31080 Pamplona
Spain

Dr. Javier Aristu
Radiotherapy Division
Department of Oncology
Clinica Universitaria de Navarra
E-31080 Pamplona
Spain

Dr. José L. Arroyo
Consultant
Department of Anesthesiology
Clinica Universitaria de Navarra
E-31080 Pamplona
Spain

Dr. Ignacio Azinovic
Radiotherapy Division
Department of Oncology
Clinica Universitaria de Navarra
E-31080 Pamplona
Spain

Dr. José L. Beguiristain
Consultant
Department of Orthopedic Surgery
and Traumatology
Clinica Universitaria de Navarra
E-31080 Pamplona
Spain

Dr. José M. Berián
Consultant
Department of Urology
Clinica Universitaria de Navarra
E-31080 Pamplona
Spain

Luther W. Brady, MD
Professor and Chairman
Hahnemann University
Department of Radiation Oncology
and Nuclear Medicine
Broad & Vine, Mail Stop 200
Philadelphia, PA 19102-1192
USA

Dr. Felipe A. Calvo
Director and Consultant
Radiotherapy Divsion
Department of Oncology
Clinica Universitaria de Navarra
E-31080 Pamplona
Spain

Dr. José Cañadell
Consultant
Department of Orthopedic Surgery
and Traumatology
Clinica Universitaria de Navarra
E-31080 Pamplona
Spain

Dr. Francisco Carrascosa
Consultant
Department of Anesthesiology
Clinica Universitaria de Navarra
E-31080 Pamplona
Spain

Dr. Fernando de la Fuente
Consultant
Department of Gynecology
Clinica Universitaria de Navarra
E-31080 Pamplona
Spain

Lluis Escudé, PhD
Medical Physics Section
Radiotherapy Division
Department of Oncology
Clinica Universitaria de Navarra
E-31080 Pamplona
Spain

Dr. Rafael Garcia-Tapia
Consultant
Department of Otorhinolaryngology
Clinica Universitaria de Navarra
E-31080 Pamplona
Spain

Dr. José L. Hernández
Consultant
Department of Surgery
Clinica Universitaria de Navarra
E-31080 Pamplona
Spain

Dr. Jesús Herreros
Consultant
Department of Cardiovascular
and Thoracic Surgery
Clinica Universitaria de Navarra
E-31080 Pamplona
Spain

Dr. Matias Jurado
Department of Gynecology
Clinica Universitaria de Navarra
E-31080 Pamplona
Spain

Dr. Rafael Llorens
Consultant
Department of Cardiovascular
and Thoracic Surgery
Clinica Universitaria de Navarra
E-31080 Pamplona
Spain

Dr. David Ortiz de Urbina
Radiotherapy Division
Department of Oncology
Clinica Universitaria de Navarra
E-31080 Pamplona
Spain

Dr. Fernando Pardo
Consultant
Department of Surgery
Clinica Universitaria de Navarra
E-31080 Pamplona
Spain

Dr. Manuel Santos
Radiotherapy Division
Department of Oncology
Clinica Universitaria de Navarra
E-31080 Pamplona
Spain

Dr. José M. Serra
Consultant
Department of Reconstructive
and Plastic Surgery
Clinica Universitaria de Navarra
E-31080 Pamplona
Spain

Dr. Luis Sierrasesúmaga
Consultant
Pediatric Oncology Unit
Department of Pediatrics
Clinica Universitaria de Navarra
E-31080 Pamplona
Spain

Dr. Enrico Tangco
Radiotherapy Division
Department of Oncology
Clinica Universitaria de Navarra
E-31080 Pamplona
Spain

Dr. Vicente Vanaclocha
Consultant
Neurosurgery Division
Clinica Universitaria de Navarra
E-31080 Pamplona
Spain

Dr. Carlos Villas
Consultant
Department of Orthopedic Surgery
and Traumatology
Clinica Universitaria de Navarra
E-31080 Pamplona
Spain

Dr. Juan Voltas
Consultant
Department of Surgery
Clinica Universitaria de Navarra
E-31080 Pamplona
Spain

Dr. Gerardo Zornoza
Consultant
Department of Surgery
Clinica Universitaria de Navarra
E-31080 Pamplona
Spain

Dr. Javier Zudiare
Consultant
Department of Urology
Clinica Universitaria de Navarra
E-31080 Pamplona
Spain

MR

Medical Radiology

Diagnostic Imaging and Radiation Oncology

Series Editors:
L. W. Brady, M. W. Donner, H.-P. Heilmann, F. Heuck

This series recognizes the demand for an international state-of-the-art account of the developments reflecting the progress in the radiological sciences. Each volume conveys an overall picture of a topical theme so that it can be used as a reference work without taking recourse to other volumes.

The contents of the volumes concentrate on new and accepted developments in a manner appropriate for review by physicians engaged in the practice of radiology.

Springer-Verlag
Berlin
Heidelberg
New York
London
Paris
Tokyo
Hong Kong
Barcelona
Budapest

G. E. Laramore, University of Washington, Seattle, WA (Ed.)

Radiation Therapy of Head and Neck Cancer

1989. XII, 237 pp. 123 figs.
Hardcover ISBN 3-540-19360-X

J.H. Anderson, The Johns Hopkins University, Baltimore, MD (Ed.)

Innovations in Diagnostic Radiology

1989. XIII, 213 pp. 144 figs. some in color.
Hardcover ISBN 3-540-19093-7

R. R. Dobelbower Jr., Toledo, OH (Ed.)

Gastrointestinal Cancer

Radiation Therapy

1990. XV, 301 pp. 76 figs. 90 tabs.
Hardcover ISBN 3-540-50505-9

E. Scherer, C.Streffer, University of Essen; **K.-R. Trott,** London (Eds.)

Radiation Exposure and Occupational Risks

1990. XI, 150 pp. 32 figs. 55 tabs.
Hardcover ISBN 3-540-51174-1

S. E. Order, The Johns Hopkins University, Baltimore, MD; **S. S. Donaldson,** Stanford University, Stanford, CA

Radiation Therapy of Benign Diseases

A Clinical Guide

1990. VIII, 214 pp. 103 tabs.
Hardcover ISBN 3-540-50901-1

R. Sauer, University of Erlangen-Nürnberg, Erlangen (Ed.)

Interventional Radiation Therapy Techniques – Brachytherapy

1991. XII, 388 pp. 193 figs. 162 tabs.
Hardcover ISBN 3-540-52465-7

E. Scherer, C. Streffer, University of Essen; **K.-R. Trott,** Medical College of London (Eds.)

Radiopathology of Organs and Tissues

1991. X, 496 pp. 156 figs. 56 tabs.
Hardcover ISBN 3-540-19094-5

M. Rotman, C. J. Rosenthal, State University of New York, NY (Eds.)

Concomitant Continuous Infusion Chemotherapy and Radiation

1991. XIV, 304 pp. 42 figs.
Hardcover ISBN 3-540-52545-9

E. K. Lang, Louisiana State University, New Orleans, LA (Ed.)

Radiology of the Upper Urinary Tract

1991. IX, 370 pp. 418 figs. 14 tabs.
Hardcover ISBN 3-540-52546-7